MARATHON MAN

MY LIFE, MY FATHER'S STROKE AND RUNNING 35 MARATHONS IN 35 DAYS

Tivoli Publishing
House

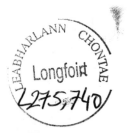

**Tivoli Publishing
House**

www.marathonman.co
Copyright © Alan Corcoran 2021

All photos © Alan Corcoran and Darren Doheny
unless otherwise stated

First Published in the Republic of Ireland in 2021
by Tivoli Publishing House

A CIP catalogue record for this book is available
from the British Library

ISBN (paperback) 978-1-8383650-0-4

This book is dedicated to my father, Milo, who taught me not to be afraid of taking a shot at goal, to my mother, Marie, for instilling thoughtfulness and care, and to my brother, Evan, for inspiring my sporting pursuits: three concrete foundation blocks of my story.

CONTENTS

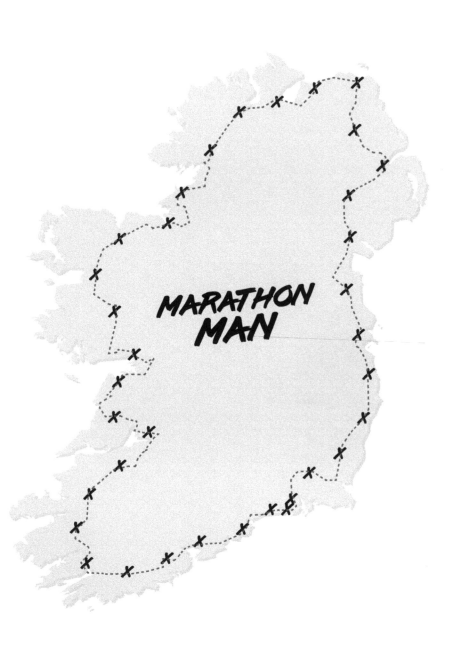

MARATHON MAN

PREFACE

In 2011 my dad, Milo Corcoran, returned to Waterford after a UEFA meeting in Switzerland. Feeling unusually tired, he took a midday nap to recuperate from the early start and long hours of travelling. He awoke in a panic, his vision suddenly impaired, one side of his body stiff, and the room spinning around him. Dad couldn't get out of bed and when he tried to drink his bedside water he nearly choked, unable to swallow.

He had just turned 60 but found himself knocking on death's door, without warning, experiencing a debilitating stroke. He was lucky he had left his phone beside him and just about managed to phone my mother, Marie, for help. He was rushed to Waterford Regional Hospital. My family's worst fears were coming to life. The best result hoped for at that point was merely survival with a daunting, slow, uphill slog to try to regain a semblance of independence.

This bombshell incident was a catalyst moment for me, then a 20-year-old Dublin Institute of Technology (DIT) Town Planning student. Although I had an acute awareness of death at that stage, I hadn't given much thought to my parents' mortality. I didn't think I needed to concern myself with the possibility of their death until they were in their eighties or became seriously ill. Dad's unexpected stroke punched me full force in the gut and the harsh reality ignited a fire under me.

Although the dream of running a lap of Ireland had been increasingly bouncing around in my head, I lacked a real incentive to take the leap and commit. After Dad's stroke, I felt compelled to do something positive. I had to make my family proud while I still could.

I needed to at least try for my pie-in-the-sky aspiration. I wanted to flip the negative incident on its head, creating an experience of a lifetime – one Dad could be an integral part of.

Motivated to grab life by the horns and take action after my dad's stroke, I set about moving the first pivotal inches towards my goal of running thirty-five back-to-back marathons as he set about recovering from his stroke. We would struggle along, on our own unique and individual challenges, supporting one another over the hurdles that came our way.

The 1,500-kilometre ultra-endurance run generated over €15,000 in charitable donations. Thanks to the support of our loved ones and the Irish community, we had the privilege of handing a large cheque to the Irish Heart Foundation, supporting their 'Act F.A.S.T.' stroke awareness campaign. We also donated to the National Rehabilitation Hospital (NRH), supporting their stroke and brain injury unit. Lastly, we contributed to the Football Village of Hope. This was a peacebuilding charity my dad helped establish, which brought Israeli and Palestinian children together, breaking down barriers, through the beautiful game.

There were lots of reasons to pursue the notion of circumnavigating Ireland on foot. To the forefront, was raising money for worthy causes. Before setting off, I told the *Irish Examiner*, 'If I don't raise enough money and hit my target, but complete the run; the challenge would still be a failure in my eyes.' Despite my all-or-nothing attitude, charitable donations failed to come close to my aspirations of €35,000, which tied in with the target of 35 marathons in 35 consecutive days.

Failing to meet the fundraising target never sat well with me.

I still have not given up hope on at least getting closer to the initial goal. Continuing in that direction, 10% of proceeds from the sale of this book will go to my two childhood sports clubs, Tramore AFC and Ferrybank AC, to contribute towards the development of the next generation of sports enthusiasts.

The run was one of my proudest endeavours and sometimes I still can't believe I attempted it. The idea wasn't imagined from thin air – I'm not that creative! I was inspired by similar feats by Eddie Izzard, Terry Fox, Dean Karnazes, Gerry Duffy and Ken Whitelaw. They in turn drew on inspiration from others when they set off on their running challenges. I would take immense satisfaction if sharing my story could continue the chain reaction and inspire others. It has been arduous spilling my guts on these pages. It would be worth the effort, if it encouraged even one person to dust off and try again, or improve their health, or chase a passion in life. Little baby steps, when taken consistently, can culminate in something massive. I hope you can draw from that and apply it to your own life.

I also hope my story can raise some awareness regarding strokes. It is vital to get emergency medical assistance if you come across someone with the signs of a stroke:

F – Face

Has their face fallen on one side? Can they smile?

A – Arms

Can they raise both of their arms and keep them there?

S – Speech

Is their speech slurred?

T – Time

To call 999 if you see the signs of a stroke.

Stroke is Ireland's third biggest killer, but hundreds of lives could be saved each year if more people knew the signs. A stroke destroys 2 million brain cells every minute. Response time is of the utmost importance – not only for the survival of the sufferer but also for the quality of life they might hope to experience after the damage is caused. If you suspect someone is having a stroke, please act F.A.S.T. and call 999.

INTRODUCTION

When introducing me, my friends tend to lead with the lap of Ireland run. After the usual prolonged and bewildered stare, the person asks, 'Are you alright in the head?' Then I'm inevitably asked, 'Why on earth would you do that to yourself?' before usually being asked, 'How, in the name of Jaysus, did you do all that?'

WHY

I'll leave my mental state for you to judge after reading this book, but *why* is essential to the story. If I hadn't been certain about my reasons for doing it, there would be no chance I'd have been able to consistently drag my arse out of bed at the crack of dawn to train, come hail, rain or shine. There would be no chance I'd have run thousands of hours on my own, plodding around the Phoenix Park in Dublin or on the roads at home in Waterford.

The initial spark of motivation, excitement and enthusiasm

can wane, or at least fluctuate. Some days running through a storm was the last thing I wanted to do. In team sports or group classes, you're held accountable by others, your team, your coach, friends and positive peer pressure. One or all of those gets you out the door and makes you show up and work when you feel lazy. This run was my brainwave, and its success or failure ultimately hinged on me, with nobody to hold me to account but myself, so I had to be sure of the reasons I was putting myself through this.

Those training sessions were usually followed by college lectures, dissertation writing and, often, my part-time job as a hotel dish-scrubber. It wasn't the typical student lifestyle, or for the faint-hearted. It didn't feel like a sacrifice, though. With a strong sense of purpose, I was stubbornly steadfast, in what was an extremely ambitious – and foolish – plan for a novice distance runner to consider.

The *why* was a result of twenty years of life experience – some positive and some negative – that finally culminated in the magical moment of certainty, when I thought to myself, *Fuck it! Let's just go for this. What have you truly got to lose, Al?*

I'll be exploring the incidents that led to the tipping point of cast-iron certainty. These moments were bits of tinder added to a pile and when my dad suffered the stroke, this was the unwanted but necessary spark for ignition. Inaction was no longer an option. I had to swing back at life for punching Dad – and as a consequence me – flat to the floor. If I didn't, I'd have to live knowing in my heart that I let us be beaten and just took it. Nobody else would know or care if I didn't take action, as it was just a whimsical notion in my thick head. However, *I* would know if I cowered away from the challenge. I couldn't be having that. If I'm going down, I'm going down swinging, not raising a white flag.

I was a runner – a failed sprinter no less – and running seemed the best outlet to vent my fear, fury and sadness, and create a positive focus. I knew sprinting wouldn't raise any money for good causes, so I needed to think bigger – much bigger. I became obsessed with the idea of running around Ireland, a marathon at a time, so I pursued this off-piste ambition of mine with vigour.

HOW

Once I had my reasons solidified in my mind, *how* was less essential. There's certainly wisdom in the sayings 'where there's a will, there's a way' and 'he who has a why to live can bear almost any how.' My father's difficult road to recovery was in contrast with the lightning speed of the stroke. Although my running challenge would not come close to the problems he would have to endure, we followed a similar how-to manual.

We both needed a problem-solving optimistic attitude to find ways to overcome life's inevitable complications. We needed to do our best to lean into the wind when it blew at its strongest against us, putting our heads down and making persistent small daily effort towards our daunting goals. Some steps were so small they seemed invisible. On rare days, some steps seemed like monumental leaps forward. It was all about being relentless. With grim persistence and determination, we would find out what we were truly made of.

ONE:

FAMILY AND FORMATIVE YEARS

MILO

In the seventies my parents, Marie and Milo, met at the Celtic Squash Club, in Waterford City. After getting married, they had my brother, Evan, and then me eight years later.

My dad was born in Dublin but his Granny, Katie, and Aunt, Nan, raised him on their farm in Clogga, Mooncoin, County Kilkenny. He dropped out of Waterford's De La Salle secondary school early to find work. He found his way into furniture sales, later becoming a sales representative for Heineken where he spent most of his career.

Having been raised in Kilkenny and lived most of his life in Waterford, he loved hurling and even got his teeth knocked out playing it, but his primary passion in life was soccer. I often pondered, while observing him at matches or in the sitting room watching a game together, how someone could care so much. I don't mean just about football or hurling, or his team winning. I mean anything. The game was like a life-or-death battle. It takes a hell of a lot to move me off centre and get me fired up over anything, but he'd be enthralled and enthused with pure passion and love for the sports. It was a sight to behold when those Manchester United or Waterford hurling tinted glasses were on, and his team could do no wrong. I got many a playful 'Ah feck off!' when I'd try to engage him rationally about the blatant foul by Paul Scholes or John Mullane, that was called up by 'that blind bollocks of a referee'. There was no talking sense into him in those moments. The ever-passionate Davy Fitzgerald effing and blinding up the sideline springs to mind as a comparison, during match time.

Although Dad provided for us by working as a sales rep, he managed to pursue his passion for football in his spare time, with my Mam's support. Supporting Waterford Football Club in the seventies, he drove all over the country, cramming players into his car to get them to matches. From the supporter's club, Dad transitioned to become part of the club's management board. Later, he even became the club's Chairman in the eighties. This progression led to his involvement with the Football Association of Ireland (FAI), being Waterford's club representative on the League Committee in the eighties and nineties. He devoted much of his time to football administration. His commitment was rewarded, eventually getting elected as Vice President of the FAI. This term was followed by being selected as FAI President in 2001, during a tumultuous and memorable period in Irish football. This stretch saw Ireland beat the Netherlands in Lansdowne Road, to qualify for the World Cup in Korea and Japan, with the subsequent infamous Roy Keane departure from Saipan.

During his time with the FAI, my dad was a member of the UEFA Youth and Amateur Football Committee, chaired the FAI's International Committee and had a significant influence on the creation of the Setanta Sports Cup. The Setanta Sports Cup was a cross-border competition, between League of Ireland clubs, from the Republic of Ireland, and Irish League clubs, from Northern Ireland. He was proud to be the tournament's Chairman from its inception in 2005, playing a small role in trying to improve relations between the north and south of the island.

Dad's Setanta Sports Cup experience came in handy when assisting his friend Ophir Zardok to create the Football Village of Hope in 2008. These summer camps gave Israeli and Palestinian kids a unique chance to meet each other, in an attempt to break the cycle of segregation and distrust. Dad's face would light up telling me about the barriers he observed falling during his time at the camps. The kids would make mincemeat of each other initially, but prejudiced squabbles subsided, with a few games together creating respect and friendship.

MARIE

My mam grew up in the seaside town of Tramore, County Waterford. She did well in school and worked to get her degree in biomedical science in Cork. Then, she devoted her entire working career to being a laboratory technician, in the haematology lab in Waterford Regional Hospital.

Mam selflessly devoted herself to supporting her family, ensuring we had our wants and needs met. Not only did she care for me, my brother and Dad, she devoted a lot of her time and energy to looking after elderly relations too. She's as reliable, thoughtful and hardworking as they come. She's also the sensible voice of reason when it comes to risk-taking, especially when the safety and security of her boys are at stake – the poster woman Irish mammy through and through!

It's beyond me how my mam juggled all her responsibilities: a full-time career, caregiving duties, meal prepping and lifts for school, training sessions, matches and competitions. This was even more impressive because Dad would regularly be away for a weekend here, a week there or even longer, with his football commitments, home and abroad. Still, with so much on her plate, Mam somehow managed to complete a part-time biomedical science master's degree in her fifties to boot. It speaks volumes of her heart and work ethic.

Mam's life may not have been as unique as my dad's – going from farm to board room, travelling the world for his hobby/ job – but it was equally inspirational. The time and devotion my mother put towards family and education and the value she placed on them hugely impacted my development. That is why family is first in my story.

EVAN

Finally, there's my big brother, Evan. Ev was always someone I could look up to. With eight years' age gap, he was stronger, faster and smarter than me growing up. He still beats me up the odd time even now!

Fortunately, he was well behaved at school, which worked in my favour. His reputation meant I was in the good books from day one, which took the pressure off for first impressions and set the standard for me to adhere to going forward. There was a clear example to follow, exam results to try to better and medal tallies to try and outdo.

Evan was a great training partner in the backyard too – although it never felt like training, just playing. He would teach me new football skills, often running rings around me. More important than the football tricks, were the lessons in getting roughed up (although he might say I was diving). These hours on hours out the back instilled a degree of toughness in me from an early age. It taught me to get up, get on with it and keep trying. There was no sympathy from Ev if he steamrolled through me, just encouragement in a brotherly fashion to persist in my doomed pursuit against him.

'Get up will ya, you're grand!' or 'You're never going to score sat on your arse, are ya?'

My success rate against him was dismal. I knew getting up would likely end in me falling for his tricks again or getting bashed down by what he called a 'fair shoulder'. Nonetheless, down and up I would continue until one of our parents would call us in for dinner; simple, fun times.

One time, when babysitting me, we took turns holding the settee cushion to practise our boxing. Somehow, Evan missed the enormous soft target and clocked me straight in the eye.

'You moved it! You alright, Al?'

'I didn't! You just punched me in the face,' I laughed.

'Shit, Mam will kill us when she gets back and sees a black eye. Get some ice.'

'Why would she kill *us*? *You*, punched *me*, in the face,' I teased.

I squirmed with the freezing peas on my eye, as Ev laughed at my wimpy response. After about five or 10 minutes, he asked if I could feel it sore or cold anymore. I told him, no, so Ev advised me to take it off for a while. When the feeling came back to my face, he instructed me to put the ice back on. Being a child, I was curious to learn what the method to the madness was.

'Why do you do that? Put the ice on and off and then back on again?'

'Oh, no reason, I just thought it was funny seeing you squeal with the cold,' he told me, with a beaming smile.

'Fucker.'

We got the swelling down, and I never said a word … until my best man speech at his wedding, donkey's years later.

I learned a lot about losing and keeping a smile on my face despite the brotherly battering. Whether Play Station, play fighting or football, it was a scarce occasion I'd get one over. He was instilling resilience.

WHERE THE ADVENTURES BEGIN

The sense of exploration and taking on challenges without a safety net seemed to be part of my nature from the jump, metaphorically and literally.

My mother recalls that before I had even turned one, or could walk, she was baffled, repeatedly finding me smiling on the bedroom floor, even though only moments before she had securely placed me in my cot surrounded by high guard rails on all sides. This was before the days of cot cameras, so Mam made do with secretly peeping around the corner of the door, unbeknown to the reckless adventurer in the cot. To her dismay, I somehow managed to clamber my tiny body onto the edge of the railing of the cot, precariously balancing my torso on it for a split second. Before my mother could react, I threw caution to the wind, as I lumped myself like a sack of spuds onto the floor, landing any which way gravity took me. That was the mystery solved and an indication of things to come for a child that was prone to giving himself a bump or 10.

Once I got on my feet, I had ants in my pants. I was an instant runner, an easily distracted explorer and a right pain in the arse for any adult given the impossible responsibility to keep an eye on me. My reputation was so bad that my older relatives and their friends wouldn't risk taking me out for a walk a second time. 'Fool me once …' and all that. I was there one second and out of sight the next.

After a few scenarios like this, I can't blame my parents for playing it safe. Still, I was horrified to see some of my cruel toddler photos recently. There I was in one of those oppressive harnesses, being walked like an excited puppy by my brother. My mam tells me it was essential and completely justified, for my own sake and for the benefit of everyone else's nerves. My inquisitive nature, lack of any self-preservation instinct and speed off the mark, must have tested the hearts of the adults around me.

FLAT ON MY FACE FOOTBALL

Sport is something I've been heavily involved in from an early age. I feel incredibly privileged and grateful to have parents that were so supportive, encouraging and accommodating with their time and earnings. They selflessly afforded me opportunities to learn new skills, be healthy and active. They enabled me to make lifelong friends and, ultimately, to be able to say I had a happy childhood, in large part due to my participation in sports.

When I was about six, my parents thought it would be a wise move to try to tire me out a bit, constructively focus my excessive energy and get them a bit of a break from chasing me. My mother started by taking me to swimming lessons. I happily and consistently pursued it for years; Mam always keeping a watchful eye on my progress from the poolside, nattering with the other swim mammies. Around the same time, she also took me to gymnastics – or at least tried to. This attempt just resulted in me bawling my eyes out and whining, without even trying. Not the highlight of my sporting endeavours!

It was no surprise my dad was keen to encourage me to play ball. I was reluctant at first, and he failed to convince me to try training for a local club; I was content with kicking about in the garden with my brother. One Saturday night, when my parents were out for dinner together, and my brother had been left in charge, I was instructed to bed as it was my bedtime. I wanted to stay up past bedtime and watch South Park. I was only around six, and it was far from appropriate for a child of my age to be watching the show. My brother probably shouldn't have been watching it either at his age, but he was the boss for the night. He made me a proposition.

'If I leave you stay up to watch one episode, will you

promise to try football training tomorrow morning?'

'Deal,' I said, without hesitation, thinking he would forget about it and I'd have conned him into letting me stay up. He didn't forget. The next morning I was rudely awakened by Dad and Ev reminding me of the deal I had made. I must have felt some obligation to fulfil my word. Somewhat reluctantly, I went out to Tramore AFC for my first memorable training, under Paul Power. It was remarkable for the wrong reasons. All I recall was falling flat on my face when asked to try a simple ball control drill in front of the group. Needless to say, it triggered a few laughs, which Paul was quick to quash. I was encouraged for my efforts to try. Paul told me to practise at home and come back to try again. As haunting as the failure was, I wasn't deterred and had the desire to get better. I practised the move all week in the garden until I no longer tripped myself up. When I was asked to demonstrate the movement again at the next weekend's training session, I hit the nail on the head. It was a joyous feeling, and I was hooked, ending up playing for the club until I went to college in Dublin, some 10 years later.

NO MEDALS FOR FOURTH PLACE

In Ballygunner primary school, while continuing to swim and play football, I picked up Gaelic football and had my interest in athletics triggered. Somehow, I managed to mysteriously avoid hurling though, in a school and community synonymous with the sport.

I was always one of the athletic kids, winning or medalling in the school sports day each year. All was golden until fourth class when I came fourth in the prestigious 100-metre sprint. We all know there are no medals for fourth place. I was used to success; that experience of failure left an unpleasant taste in my mouth. I faced a choice after losing. Do I get upset and whine? Do I shrug it off and do nothing, likely remaining fourth or finishing lower next year? Or do I take ownership of the loss and do something about it to avoid that sinking feeling of failure next time?

I remembered failing at my first football training, working on the failed drill in solitude and sticking it to the group the next time of asking. The practice avoided the kids laughing at me the second time around. With that lesson in mind, I thought to apply the same approach. I would try to get one up on my classmates the next year, joining the local athletics club, Ferrybank AC.

Admittedly, not all my intentions were as admirable as wanting to better myself and be more competitive. A few of the boys I was friends with did athletics and promised me there were loads of nice girls at training too. At the age of 10 or so, this seemed as good a reason as any. If I beat my classmates and got some shiny medals in the process of having fun with my friends and meeting girls, then there were no downsides to this little venture of mine.

My initiative and hard work couldn't have gone better. I managed to win the 100-metres race in fifth and sixth class. I even racked up a few medals for Ferrybank AC, in the County, Munster and All-Ireland Championships. I earned a medal in the Scottish Indoor Championships too and running was becoming a large part of my persona. My initial defeat that drove me to athletics was in the rear-view. I was enjoying the fun and success, training, improving and competing. Athletics even led to my first kiss, in the warm-up area of Nenagh's corrugated iron indoor 'stadium', and meeting Mairéad, my first girlfriend and childhood sweetheart – success all round.

This was an invaluable early life lesson: sucking at something and feeling hard done by for my own failure, using the negative experience to fuel the response, and coming back stronger, more prepared for the next rodeo. Fall down five times, rise up six.

Although I was having early success in running, I hadn't had too much running ambition beyond wanting to be the fastest in my school class. The real dream in primary school was to be a full-time footballer for Manchester United. Nearly every Christmas and birthday, I wanted a football or a Ryan Giggs jersey, and my parents did their best to deliver on those occasions.

I had football training every week during the season. Every day we were allowed on the grass at school, the jumpers and lunchboxes were put down as goalposts: it was time for fun. When school and the football season were out for summer, I was off to as many football summer camps as I could get.

If I wasn't at athletics, swimming or football, I was usually endlessly kicking the ball against the wall to myself at the side of our house or doing keepie-uppies in the garden. This might seem mind-numbing to most, but I enjoyed it, imagining I was on trial at Man U, tasked to do as many kick-ups as possible or demonstrate my passing with both feet.

On weekends, I'd dribble the ball up and down Woodstown Beach, like a dog playing fetch, as my family walked and booted the ball for me to chase down and return. One winter, I didn't retrieve the new Christmas football in time. It floated into the sea, the choppy outbound tide dragging it out quickly. Dad wasn't a swimmer. The only time he experienced floating was in the Dead Sea. Because of that, this moment stands out. Despite his caution of the sea and the late December temperature, he waded in fully clothed without hesitation. He triumphantly held my beloved ball overhead, the water bobbing at chest height by the time he reached it. If that ain't love, I don't know what is!

For 'down time' then, I precariously climbed up and fell off walls and trees and often played chase on my street with a great gang of friends around the same age. My childhood was endless energy, movement and being outdoors.

TWO:

ADOLESCENCE

PREPUBESCENT OGRE

For the most part, it was sunshine and rainbows as a young kid. I did well enough in school and in sports, had friends and stayed out of trouble. It wasn't all smiles, though. I began getting acne towards the end of my primary school days. Needless to say, this generated some comments from inconsiderate kids that knocked me. I had to get braces for my messed-up mouth too. If the start of a bad skin condition wasn't enough to wipe the smile off my face, the braces certainly helped. The chunky plastic palate stuck to the roof of my mouth, creating a severe lisp, deterring me from speaking, and the metal bar across my teeth made me more self-conscious and unwilling to smile. To add insult to injury, there were days of pain every time the screws were tightened, forcing my wonky teeth closer to where they were meant to be. I felt like I was slowly transforming into a prepubescent ogre and my self-worth took a hit. My shoulders hunched a little, and my gaze lowered a fraction. In the grand scheme of things these were minor health issues to deal with, but difficult for a kid to live with nonetheless. I was singled out from the herd for the wrong reasons, adding weight on my scrawny shoulders.

I hated the braces and skin problems at the time but, in hindsight, the adversity shaped me for the better. It gave me thicker skin and more drive, with pent up pain and frustration fuelling my development. While I didn't appreciate getting comments on something I couldn't do much to change, the unpleasantness reminded me to be more considerate when speaking to others. The hard times, made me appreciate painless days more, when my mouth wasn't in agony, and my skin wasn't breaking out. Perspective can help in moments of difficulty or perceived difficulty. Things could always be worse, and most problems are temporary.

I felt awkward in my skin, but sport was an avenue to a different world. When I was playing or racing, I was just present and wasn't consumed with how visible the spots on my face were or how my crooked smile looked. I was way too busy trying to win and just having fun. Despite the growing insecurities and periods of unpleasant pain, I was still a competitive runner and footballer, better than most around me. My involvement in sports was critical, enabling me to retain some confidence and self-worth.

I may have got a 'pizza face' or 'spotty' here or there on the pitch, but the opposition rarely persisted, as I did my best to crunch the bully in the next tackle and worked in overdrive to outplay them in all aspects, making sure my enjoyment was visible. It pissed me off, for sure, but I was able to channel the negativity productively. I'd go harder, feeling I had a point to prove. I wanted to be known as the footballer or runner or swimmer – not pimple head or brace face.

TIME OF YOUR LIFE

I learned a cruel lesson about life's fragility in 2001, near the end of my primary school days. I had been to funerals of older adults, and that's what I thought happened to everyone: you live until 80 or 90 and die of old age. People are prepared and expect it, as relatives deteriorate over time. It made no sense when my friend, babysitter and neighbour, Nicole Weldon, died suddenly. She was only 15 years old and a normal, fit and healthy young girl.

We were a close little street of kids, always out playing and running about. Although Nicole was in the older group – her brother, Marc, and sister, Lauren, were my age – Nicole used to supervise jumping-off-the-swings competitions in their garden and would share new music with us – the likes of Green Day and Linkin Park.

I couldn't believe it when Mam told me what had happened, one day after picking me up from school.

'What? No! How could that be? That's not right!'

Reality hit hard at the packed funeral. I remember feeling flushed, sick and overwhelmed by the gravity of the moment, needing to take a break outside, while my dad put his arm around me. I needed air and a minute to breathe, before rejoining the mass to hear Green Day's 'Time of Your Life' play in her memory.

Nicole's unexpected death ended a significant part of my

youthful innocence. The jarring moment made me look at life differently. The experience terrified me. I realised I could die today – and so could anyone. As unjust as it was, life and time went on, but I often found and still do find myself thinking about this sudden tragedy, how unfair and unpredictable life can be at times and the importance of not taking anything for granted.

SPORTS TAKE OVER

I followed my father's and brother's footsteps into De La Salle secondary school. There I joined the football team, the Gaelic football team and represented the school in athletics. I also picked up basketball. As one of the lankiest lads in the year, I had no problem sailing onto that team. A large part of the appeal of all those school teams were those lovely few half days off school here and there – and being allowed play more.

'I can get off school *and* play sports? Sign me up! I'll play for the older age group teams too, if they'll have me.' We also had one of the longest lunch breaks in the country. I could train in the middle of the day for as many school teams as would take me, without it conflicting with after school club training commitments. It was perfect.

Athletics demanded three or four training sessions per week, usually two track sessions, a hill sprints session and circuit training. Once I was around 16, there were one or two weights sessions as well. One more session was required for football with Tramore AFC and then a match on most weekends of the season. There was a lot on my plate with schoolwork, club training, and the school sports teams, but I became proficient at juggling the demands. I was in a productive routine that I loved.

With all those sporting commitments, I decided to say goodbye to swim lifesaving classes after six years. My age restricted me from accessing the next stage of qualifications and I didn't feel like repeating until I was old enough by their standards. Even with swimming dropped, it was still a full-on schedule, but I didn't think anything of the daily routine, thinking it was normal. I was up at 07:30 a.m. for school, straight to afterschool study, 10–20-minute nap at home, training with my friends, shower, dinner with my family and bed by 11:00 p.m. Rinse and repeat like clockwork during the week. Friday night was date night – a pot of tea in O'Brien's with Mairéad – and most weekends were hanging out with friends after the morning's sport was done.

It was only later in life that I realised it was more usual for kids to sit in front of a screen after school, hang about aimlessly, or even study *after* the afterschool study. I think it's madness – children would be in school studying nine to five and would then be doing more schoolwork at home after that. That's probably why I'm not a doctor or lawyer! Still, I feel I managed to strike a more rounded existence with the right balance of school, sports, family and socialising.

MARATHON SEED PLANTED

It was when I was in secondary school that the first tiny seed was planted about marathon running. I was an avid track sprinter at this stage. The sprint group were always reluctant to partake in anything beyond 400 metres, especially the wet, mucky misery involved in the compulsory long-distance cross-country races.

Attendance was expected, to bolster the club's dominance and help lay a solid foundation of fitness for the year's sprint training. Although the sprinters dreaded the unglamorous suffering involved in going up and down muddy hills in the depths of winter, particularly against specialist distance runners, we caved to the coaches' desire and healthy peer pressure from one another to show up and compete. We trusted in the process and represented the club the best we could. Andy Hallissey, the athletics club's wise father, used to tell us sprinters that the cross-country races are like putting money in the bank. You voluntarily invested in the hardship and you were tougher for it, getting to withdraw the winter deposit with interest on the track during the height of the summer sprint season. As kids we always found his animated explanation and analogy funny but there was undoubtedly wisdom in it. There was no instant gratification here, just repeated difficult situations and small deposits of time and effort to try to ensure a win in the future.

Despite the suffering experienced during the cross-country races I competed in as an early teen, the London Marathon's spectacle seemed a different prospect altogether and piqued my interest. It was something I tuned in to most years on the BBC, wrapped in my warm cosy sleeping bag on the couch, as the sweat-drenched celebrities, werewolves and Big Bens hobbled past. Huge crowds were lining the entire route, cheering, as the commentary dipped from the elite legends like Paula Radcliffe, running at breakneck speed, to the average Joe and Jane with their own deep and personal reasons to put themselves through this epic test of endurance. I remember telling myself that I'd do *one* marathon someday, once I packed in the sprinting and no longer needed my fast-twitch muscle fibres to race. The marathon seed was planted but needed a hell of a lot of watering and time to grow.

DABBLING IN ROAD RUNNING

One outlier race I participated in, while in secondary school, was a charity school run when I was around 14 years of age. The run was 16 kilometres on the roads, from Waterford City to Tramore and back to De La Salle School. It was well beyond any random 30-minute jog around the block I would have done with my brother, but there was no fear in me.

Given the distance involved, it was restricted to senior students only. I had to make a special case for an exception to be made and blagged my way in as a junior pup. My athletics medals for the school proved enough to convince Brother Thomas that I wouldn't keel over and die. I took it as a bit of fun and an excuse to get off class, rather than trying to race it. I had to make sure that I left enough in the tank for sprint training a few hours afterwards. I did alright in the fundraiser event, nonetheless.

Believe it not, I never got near running 16 kilometres for the six years after that. I wouldn't even surpass the five-kilometre mark until I told the Irish Heart Foundation that I was running a lap of Ireland, foolishly affording myself eight months to prepare. Things changed with a bang then.

ENDURANCE

The success I was having on the track was dampened as I struggled with my worsening skin condition. I recall smashing it and qualifying to represent Ireland in the multi-events, consisting of sprint hurdles, long jump, high jump, shot putt and the 800 metres. After the qualifying competition, I should have been ecstatic but I found myself, counterintuitively, at one of my lowest points.

My only distinct memory of that day is refusing to eat out with my parents, midway through the drive home from Dublin to Waterford. Mam and Dad had made the long drive and spent the entire day cheering me on for the chance to represent our country. They just wanted to enjoy a celebratory meal together to mark the victory. To their confusion, disappointment and frustration, no doubt, I stubbornly refused the offer. As they ate in the restaurant, I curled into a protective ball on the floor behind the driver's seat. In the darkness, reeking of sweat, I was listening to a mopey Coldplay song through my headphones, with tears coming down my face. The demands of the full day's exertion probably added to the raw hormone-fuelled emotions. Prolonged and strenuous exercise has a way of stripping back the layers of even the most hardened souls, never mind a young teenage boy having a particularly bad skin day. Nobody had said anything to cause offence or upset. I'd performed excellently, achieving a big goal of mine, yet there I was weeping, struggling to cope with the anguish of my deteriorating, painful and unsightly skin condition.

As my teenage acne worsened, photographic evidence of this period of my life is scarce as I ran for cover once anyone brandished a camera. I was regularly going to the doctors, systematically going through all the medicines they would give me to cure the problem, but none had long-lasting effects. Some would make it better temporarily, getting my hopes and mood up, then I'd be dejected as the condition made a rampant return. Having spent months on one dose of tablets and failed, I'd try a new prescription that would aggravate my skin more, and so the cycle would continue. Having exhausted the safer options, we eventually landed on Roaccutane, a somewhat notorious medication. Common side effects include headaches and general aches and pains, and dry eyes, nose and throat. Serious side effects include things such as suicide, severe stomach pain, difficulty moving your arms or legs, and painful, swollen or bruised areas of the body. The scary list of severe side effects went on and on, coming with a sober warning. It was no joke, requiring regular blood tests and appointments with the dermatologist to keep track of my overall health.

The doctor thought it unlikely that I'd have the ability to do sports while undergoing treatment. I was willing to take the risk though, hoping for pain-free living and a chance of becoming more relaxed and less self-conscious. The meds made things much worse for an extended period. They created inflamed boils, like nothing I had before, mainly on my neck, but on my chest and face too. Some of these things you could pop 10 heads out of, streams of blood and gunk swirling around the shower drain, as if someone was murdering me. It was disgusting and hard to live with, but I knew the tablets were my last resort for a fix, and I had to just endure the side-effects. I remember the daily pain, Jesus, the pain caused by the stiff school uniform collar that used to make me grimace when I'd twist and turn my neck. It was physically unbearable at times. It was like being in a neck brace on bad days, turning my entire body to keep the neck as still as possible to minimise the friction on the inflamed, sensitive skin.

Seeing my physical suffering, the doctor offered to write me a note for school, to allow me to wear a round-neck t-shirt instead of the pain-inducing stiff uniform collar. That approach would have slightly reduced the physical pain but didn't outweigh the increased anxiety it would cause; a t-shirt making the angry volcanoes visible for all to see and comment on. On balance, I decided to suck up the physical pain instead, covering up my spots with my blood-stained school shirt, caps, scarfs, turtlenecks and popped polo shirt collars, at all opportunities. It passed for fashion rather than a functional disguise, and it kept my self-consciousness at bay. Without a doubt, the cheese-grater sensation of my clothing against my skin made the condition and the pain worse, but at least nobody could see, and I could absorb the constant soreness internally. It was a slog. The unyielding irritation and pain were putting me on edge and making me frustrated and irritable. It was in contrast to who I felt I was: a generally happy-go-lucky smiley kid.

Shitty skin has nothing to do with marathon running on the face of it, but, in my experience, it taught me a hell of a lot about endurance and continuing to show up. Google Dictionary defines endurance as '1The ability to endure an unpleasant or difficult process or situation without giving way. 2The capacity of something to last or to withstand wear and tear.' The condition was a significant part of my youth. It wore on me daily and

leader board. Points for the country would be won regardless of whether it was Chris or me in the medals, but we never held back in training and weren't going to start now. We wanted to beat each other and kept the pedal to the metal. Between 100 metres to go and 50 metres to go, we were neck and neck, mere hundredths of seconds separating us. Lactic acid riddled and tightening up, we were in the heat of battle.

If you haven't experienced lactic acid build-up, I'd think it difficult to imagine. This by-product builds up in your muscles if pushed hard enough and long enough, depleting them of oxygen. The higher the intensity, the more lactic acid that's created, the more intense the pain becomes and the more strenuous running gets. It is impossible to ignore.

If you're curious to feel this sensation, then warm up, stretch, and sprint flat out for just 400 metres/one lap of a track or roughly 60 seconds if you can't reach a track. Be honest and sprint hard from the word go to the finish line. You will know all about it then.

The legs will become heavier and heavier, burning, as you struggle to lift your knees with the lactic taking hold. The lungs, arms and legs are in overdrive, your brain yelling *GO!* but your body slows regardless. Now imagine, while feeling that sensation, you're facing a weighted waist-height barrier hurtling towards you, and you need to jump over it as efficiently and smoothly as possible. Testing, to say the least.

Back on the track, I was fractionally ahead of Chris, with nine hurdles cleared and only one hurdle to go. I was on pace for a personal best. Then, my leap came up short and I destroyed myself off the last barrier. My body skidded along the rough synthetic track and tore my skin. The adjacent stadium cheers immediately turned to 'oohs', as I walloped the ground. Without thought, I bounced straight back up. I was running towards the line again, although worse for wear, running purely on adrenaline and now in eighth and last place. I was pissed off that I bottled the podium finish and points for my team. Still, I was happy for Chris, who was more concerned for me when he crossed the line than he was about celebrating his medal win. I couldn't have lost to a more worthy opponent.

After the event, the coaches made a speech about the team's performance on the Irish Team bus. To my surprise, they singled out my performance. *I was last, why the fuck are they talking about me?* They emphasised the character they thought it displayed. By getting up and finishing, I got one point on our team's scoreboard. This was one more point than if I had just lain there and sulked in defeat or retreated off the track to a disqualification. To be honest, that one point never crossed my mind. There wasn't time to think. It was just an automatic reaction for me to keep going, and I thought nothing of getting up. I expected it of myself. The Irish Team coaches' tip of their hat was nice to hear, nonetheless. It restored some pride, after an otherwise embarrassing day out. I might have been a loser, but I was a loser with the right mindset and attitude at least. There's no shame in losing or getting knocked on your ass (or face in this instance), but I would be ashamed if I didn't get up and give it my all to the line. On that occasion, dead last was my all. Live, learn and move on.

That perseverance wasn't licked off the stones. It was forged mostly through the completion of tough, consistent training sessions at my local track. The training was extremely demanding, and we had to become hardened animals, completing the tasks set for us each week. I hadn't fully appreciated it at the time, but it was such a great environment to have placed myself in, instilling character traits like mental toughness, without even knowing it. It was an exciting time to be part of Ferrybank AC, with a large and successful teenage training group coached by the committed Brid and Alan Golden. We boys and girls were cleaning up shop every year at the County, Munster, and National Championships. We were making up a significant number of athletes when we were old enough to join the juvenile Irish Teams too.

Despite running being a solo endeavour, we enjoyed a supportive team atmosphere. We pushed and encouraged each other through absolute physical and mental torture. Each training session, we were being tested against the top juvenile sprinters in the country. Most of my group went on to get running scholarships in Ireland and abroad, and many went on to have senior success on the international stage. My clubmates Jessie and Thomas Barr even became Olympic sprinters!

We'd spend most of the training being kids, flirting, laughing and joking through the 15-minute warm-up, followed by 45 minutes of technique work out of the starting blocks, over the hurdles or into the sandpit. The real donkey work was left to the end – the last 15 minutes. The atmosphere would notably change at this point. There would always be apprehensiveness waiting for the coach to declare what's on the menu for the evening. Once announced, the jury would be in.

'Oh god,' someone would sigh.

'This is gonna suck balls,' from someone else.

Nerves and the heart rate would increase in anticipation of the misery we now knew was in store if we pushed ourselves – and we always did. There would be dread in the air, but we were there now, so we'd have to get through it one way or another. The switch would turn from the initial negativity.

'Come on, lads, let's go,' we'd encourage each other.

'We got this.'

'Once we get these first two runs done; we'll be over the hump.'

We'd psyche ourselves up, slapping our own legs and face, taking some deep breaths, knowing that once the first whistle sounded, there'd be no escape, with set rest times, set distances and number of repetitions to adhere to. No retreat. There would be no hiding either. Running is no team sport. You and you alone are accountable for how you perform. It is clear for you and all to see, equally matched peers in the lanes to your left and right, keeping you honest and pushing you towards the line on each sprint.

My eventual specialist event, the 400-metre hurdles, is as challenging a discipline as any to prepare for. Specialising in a shorter distance or field events, got you less painful, shorter, faster training sessions. These training sessions focused on speed and power. Specialise in the 800 metres or anything above, meant you were in the long-distance training group, running laps and hitting the road, focusing more on volume and endurance. Four hundred metres and 400-metre hurdles are the tortuous middle ground, demanding speed endurance.

Unlike the lazy feckers in the speed group, all our 400-metre group puked at some point, knackered after some hellish session, running too hard for too long. I was known for being particularly bad for this, repeatedly pushing myself to breaking point. Hating this side effect, I thought it was my diet first, so I'd try to eat less between lunchtime and training, eat further from practice, or eat something different, lighter. Instead of pasta on the track though, I'd be dry heaving nothing or just water. Having tried to address it and failed, I just accepted sometimes I'm going to puke, and it won't be pleasant. I didn't let the fact hold me back from pushing to the line each time. The odd time, I'd be retching between running reps, with only four or five out of the six runs complete.

'How many recovery minutes left, Billy?' I'd shout to my training partner, who was walking back to the start line, as I was hunching over the advertisement hoarding which lined the side of the track.

'Two minutes, Al, you alright?'

'Just my sandwich from lunch. I'll see you on the start line.'

The call from coach Alan would come.

'10 seconds!'

My toe would be on the line, heart going like the clappers, telling myself *one more, that's all, all or nothing!* When the whistle shrieked, I'd be off flat out, racing my friends again.

Completing these testing training sessions demanded a hugely positive mindset, resilience, perseverance, determination and encouragement, both from our own internal self-talk dialogue, and friends, who were right there in survival mode too.

We were hardy nutters, but the method was working. We were winning, so we were back for more pain each week. Strange, nobody ever forced us to go or do anything we didn't want. You were free to walk off the track at any point in time, but we didn't. Despite our young age, we decided to be there. We chose not to quit, fighting the natural response of most sensible people to avoid scenarios of extreme discomfort. We quite literally ran towards what we feared, the deep waters of the intensely painful fatigue. When you think about it, training was pretty masochistic. We derived a twisted satisfaction in the process of getting to perceived limits and continuing anyway. We did what many couldn't even imagine, as they would have resigned from the track before getting to the level of discomfort we learned to cope with. We individually controlled our dials of intensity and whacked it recklessly to full, pushing to failure. Recovering and rebuilding our bodies to be more robust, all to repeat the process, forging seemingly bulletproof bodies *and* minds. This hard work gave us all the edge and earned us the right to have self-belief on race day.

It was damn intense in hindsight but strangely normal for us all. Balls to the wall and flat-out racing, lungs at capacity and muscles burning. That was just the first sprint usually out of about six. We'd then have to tell ourselves to hold on for dear life, forcing ourselves to keep that effort up, as the shockwaves of pain and suffering ramped up with each additional run. Finally, we'd make it to the end. The track would be strewn with teenagers, some in the foetal position, some on their hands and knees. Others would be on their backs with their legs raised at 90 degrees. That just leaves the pukers, making all sorts of noises as far from the group as they could get before the inevitable.

From our perspective, the sole goal was to get faster and stronger physically. We trusted the coaches and knuckled down to get the necessary work done while enjoying each other's company. As a consequence of chasing speed gains, we developed an unbreakable spirit to push on through any agony. There is great strength and power to be taken from repeatedly forcing your body and mind way into that darkness and soldiering through regardless.

THREE:

COLLEGE

RUNNING WITH THE BIG BOYS

I applied for college athletics scholarships across Ireland. I was
hoping my few modest international races and 30 plus All-Ireland
medals would show enough promise to justify some support. In
the end, I got enough Leaving Cert points in 2008 to study my
second choice: Town Planning in DIT. As I had just won gold in the
under-19 All-Ireland 400-metre hurdles, the college interviewed
me for their sports funding programme. I got rejected, as they
decided it best to spend their cash investing in other athletes.
Fresh off a national gold medal, this vote of no confidence took
the wind out of my sails. It was demoralising for a minute, but I
tried to flip it and use it to drive my training forward. That's my
MO and always has been. If I can do something, then get on with
it. If not, then try not to waste any more energy on it and move on.
In the wise words of my dad, 'fuck 'em!' If someone was trying to
pressure him, that's what he'd say. They would have to wait until

he was good and ready himself. Or if someone wasn't willing to assist him, 'fuck 'em!' The train was leaving with or without them. I'd just have to accept the rejection and crack on with my studies and athletics ambitions without DIT's financial support.

I had chosen to study in Dublin because most of the best track athletes trained there. My brother had studied in Dublin too, and I had heard good things. At 17, I craved a move, to grow up and try to become more independent. I felt I needed to move to advance. My training group was almost entirely dismantled by then, friends departing Waterford to study and train all over the country and the world.

I sought out Jim Kidd, the former coach of David Gillick. Gillick was training under Nick Dakin in England but had learned his trade under Mr Kidd. David had just won the 400-metres gold medal for Ireland, in the European Indoor Championships. It was a massive achievement for an Irish sprinter. I remember the goosebumps, the Irish pride and sheer joy watching him succeed and celebrating on the BBC. He was like a mad man possessed, pumping his fists with his green and white jester hat on and tricolour aloft. All his hard graft paid off in that moment of glory.

It seemed a smart move to try to get in with Jim's senior sprint group at Dundrum South Dublin (DSD) Athletics Club. I had some potential and Mr Kidd welcomed me into his small, close-knit group, which trained out of Irishtown Stadium, in Ringsend. There was Jonathan Miller, who'd run 52 seconds for the 400-metre hurdles, and Nick Hogan, who'd run under 48 seconds for the 400-metres. These guys were winning senior All-Ireland medals. They were representing the country at senior level too. That's not to mention, David Connolly and Claire Bergin, two Olympic bobsledding powerhouses. It was a step up. I felt I put myself exactly where I needed to be if I were to succeed, training with some of the island's best sprint athletes.

It was strange at first. In Waterford, I was used to finding coaches herding 100 crazy kids like cats. In Dublin, there were just 10 athletic adults a few years my senior maturely conversing. It was a totally different training method to Ferrybank AC too. There are no shortcuts to progress in athletics, and it required toughness to keep up with the big boys, but it wasn't as intense as my days with Ferrybank. Every training run at home in Waterford was like an All-Ireland final, literally racing the best in the country of my age. We'd go like a flash in the first run and then try to repeat the effort for the rest, slowly fading. Under Mr Kidd it was a much more measured approach, with set times that he'd expect us to hit on each run. It was more about steady and consistent sprinting, rather than constant racing. We'd run in a group, taking turns pacing, rather than each sprinter lining up in their own lane on the staggered race lines. Although it was different, I liked having to adapt, showing up to the track with something to prove, managing to keep up with the pace and mixing with the seniors.

However, before lacing my sprint spikes, donning my Lycra shorts and pulling up my compression socks, I made sure to enjoy DIT's fresher's week – and the week before too, just for good measure. We were on the lash for about two weeks straight, until I was bleary-eyed and down to counting pennies. I was all in for the session, but when it came time to stop, I stopped. I was off the hooch, for what I had hoped would be a pivotal year ahead in my sprint progression.

This complete about-turn in my lifestyle came as a great surprise to the entire student apartment block. They'd quickly become accustomed to seeing me and my Waterford friend Rob Keller, knocking on doors and rounding up the troops for a fun night out. You could argue that I tended to enjoy myself a bit too much when I was on my training break. We sprinters were given about six weeks off to let our hair down after the summer race season. When training resumed for the dark winter's donkey work, we'd voluntarily put ourselves on the straight and narrow until the next six-week break, a year later. I found the switch in mentality easy. When one-hundredth of a second can lose a race or result in missing out on a qualifying time, a two-week drinking ban just before the competition doesn't cut it.

There is no hiding place as a runner, whether in training or in a race. Pursuing competitive athletics requires extreme and continued strict discipline for 10.5 months of the year. You might scrape football training hungover or even play a match, the sub-par performance masked by teammates, but you won't be long in getting found out if you're told to sprint 10 x 200-metres, maintaining 28–30 second times, taking just two minutes walking recovery between them. These lessons in discipline meant my tools were sharpened when it came time to prep for the 35 consecutive marathons. I knew I could turn on the discipline when needed. When the time came for marathon training, there was no significant change required. I'd just switch from the sprint poison to the ultra-running poison, 'ultra' referring to any foot race beyond the traditional full-marathon distance of 42.2 kilometres.

Being a runner was a bit of a lonely existence for a 17-year-old first-year college student, especially with it being my first extended period away from home. Once I stopped drinking, there was only so many sober nights out I felt like doing. Trying to recover for the next intense training session after being out half the night is ill-advised, even while on the dry. It's just not possible to be at your best while sleep-deprived, so even sober nights out were limited, which isolated me from mainstream college life.

I shared a student flat with five other freshers in Rialto, on the city's inner southside. At first, all were on their best behaviour making good impressions. After some months, the veils started slipping, and I'd often find people smoking with my flatmates in the shared kitchen and living space. When my training kicked off, they respected me asking them to smoke outside on the balcony but then forgot about it once they got comfortable. After repeated pleas, I just retreated to my bedroom away from the smoke. That's where I spent a large part of my time when I wasn't commuting, training, or in lectures. On weekends, the entire apartment building emptied as all the students headed home. I needed to stay in Dublin on my own though, as one of our main training sessions was hill sprints on a Saturday morning, in Kilbogget Park, Loughlinstown. I'd spend over an hour getting there on public transport. We'd have a bit of a chat and then get warmed up, before getting down to serious business.

These were always testing sessions. Jim liked these tests, as did I. One night under the track's floodlights, I told him I'd played a football match for DIT in the morning, so I couldn't anticipate hitting the target sprint times. He didn't like me making excuses in advance and believed I could hit the times regardless. As we approached the start line, he made a surprise announcement.

'Alan, you're leading and setting the pace for the group – unless you don't want to?'

'I'm game, Jim.'

I rarely led and usually tucked behind the senior internationals. I was bricking it, but the added pressure of not wanting to let Jim or the group down helped me pull it out of the bag, shocking myself.

Another night we completed our five sprints as prescribed by the monthly training plan, emptying the tank for the final 150 metres on Coach's instructions. We all dropped to our hands and knees, sticking to the frosty track once we crossed the line, steam rising off our wearied bodies.

'I want you all back to the 200-metre start in two minutes. One more run,' Jim declared. He offered me an out, as the young pup of the senior group. 'Alan, it's optional for you.'

'I'm good,' I said, throwing a thumbs up, as I struggled to my feet – far from good but making my way to the start line anyway. I wanted to progress, and I didn't want to be the weak link or get special treatment for my youth. I mightn't have been the most talented or fastest but tell me when to go, and I'll happily give what's in the tank.

Back on the Saturday hills, when I could breathe and walk again and had wiped the puke from my lips, it was time for the cooldown, bus, walk and Luas home. All in, it took the guts of nearly four hours to get the beneficial training effects of 10 focused minutes of sprint work. That gives an insight into the time commitment required and the pain threshold that's standard to bear in these types of gruelling sessions. It's no place for a weak mindset or a lack of determination.

With my hard work done for the day, I'd be back to the empty flat by lunchtime, to hang about, waiting for the rest of the students to return from their hometowns on Sunday night. At the time, I felt sacrificing my student social life and trips home to friends and family would be worth it, to compete at the National Senior Championships. I was working on and hoping for a breakthrough year and was doing what I felt necessary to achieve it.

Training times indicated I'd made the desired progress. I should have been capable of challenging for a National Senior Championship bronze medal, with a respectable 54-55 something second 400-metre-hurdles time. The hard work and sacrifice didn't pay off for me, though. The race clock kept displaying times a second or two slower than my previous years, rather than the forecast second or two faster. My coach and I were baffled by it and thought it must be a head problem, more than a lungs or legs problem.

Accustomed to competing for gold, I was demoralised to be making up numbers in my first year competing at senior level. I came home in seventh place, way off the pace, in the All-Ireland final, with a sluggish 58-second time. The infamous athletics phrase, 'next year' was echoed by everyone, as I left Santry Stadium with my head slumped.

EDDIE IZ RUNNING

Amidst the disappointment of my underperformance that summer, the marathon seed received a downpour of nourishing rainfall. One day my brother had called me to his bedroom, thinking I might be interested in a show he was watching on TV. This seemingly nothing moment was responsible for sparking off the 35-marathon concept in my head. It's bonkers the things that can profoundly impact your life, the moments that can stand out amongst all the memories.

I sat on the carpet beside his bed and, together, we watched the BBC documentary *Eddie Iz Running*. It was about an unfit 47-year-old doing a running challenge for charity. The face wasn't familiar to me but the voiceover explained that it was the comedian Eddie Izzard. The name didn't ring any bells either. Still, the intro indicated that Eddie wasn't a *runner* runner. The show would be about a celebrity pushing themselves for entertainment and raising money for charity.

The camera showed Eddie Izzard rocking up to the Olympic Medical Institute to get assessed before starting the endurance event. With an average middle-aged body, Eddie was sauntering in to discuss the challenge with a leading sports consultant, Dr Mike Loosemore. Eddie starts by telling the consultant that the plan is to run around the UK.

'The route is about 1,000 miles,' Eddie informs the doctor.

'That's a huge undertaking. What's your running history,' the health expert enquires.

'Well, when I was a kid, I ran about a bit in the playground. Erm. I'm just. I'm just. Well, I haven't done. I kind of. I think I should run. I think I'm designed for running.'

'Sorry to go back,' the consultant interrupts, 'as far as running's concerned, how much *actual* running training have you done?'

'I've done about two weeks training,' Eddie admits while pulling a face which says *I know I'm blagging it.*

'So, we haven't got 20 years of running experience up to this point?'

'No.'

'How long have you got before you do the run?'

'Eh, going in four weeks.'

The answer took Dr Loosemore by surprise. There was an awkward pause.

'Is that right?' the doc enquires with astonishment, now turned to face Eddie's team, standing out of camera shot.

Dr Loosemore gave up on Eddie and hoped one of the entourage would give a more sensible response. Someone might end the joke and say the comedian is only having him on for the sake of the cameras, but the team confirmed it was only four weeks until the running challenge was set to begin. The doctor took notes, as the rest of the room laughed. 'Janey Mackers' is what I imagined the notes read.

'Am I doing things wrong?' Eddie jokes.

'I thought we had nine months,' Dr Loosemore explains, as any sensible person would think.

'No, I don't want to do the nine months thing.'

The out-of-condition comedian was then shown hooked up to a machine like a lab rat, plodding shirtless on the treadmill for full visual effect. As we're shown Eddie gasping for air, ex-Olympian and Director of the Olympic Medical Institute, Professor Greg Whyte, confirms that the undertaking is 'ludicrous'.

All the expert assessments indicated there wasn't a hope in hell Eddie would complete the task – one thousand miles with little training. Not only expert opinion but common sense leaned strongly towards imminent failure too. The blistered journey wasn't pretty, and some days it took Eddie over 10 hours to cover the day's 42.2 kilometres. Ev and I watched, waiting for Eddie to quit as Eddie's body broke down, now roaring in agony on our TV screen as the physio poked and prodded.

'Eddie can't continue like that, surely?' I asked my brother.

'Seems impossible, alright. It's not even the halfway point, is it?'

Nevertheless, Eddie feckin' did it anyway, despite the odds and suffering, defiantly trudging through 43 marathons in 51 days, raising more than £200,000 for Sports Relief in the process. We were left blown away by what we had witnessed – sheer unrelenting perseverance.

Full of inspiration after seeing the TV show, I went for a slow five-kilometre jog the next morning with Ev. We were both mystified by what the completely unfit Eddie had accomplished. Age, appearance and lack of meaningful training signalled to my brain that it would not be possible. I couldn't quite correlate how Eddie was putting one foot in front of the other over such a mind-boggling distance. My calves and lungs were feeling the pressure of the five-kilometre jog, and I was a seasoned athlete. It just didn't make sense. *Fair play!* I thought.

It was just a fleeting interest at the time. After our little enthusiastic road run and debrief over family breakfast, I didn't put any further thought into Eddie's odyssey for another year or so. I was still a college sprinter, training up to seven times a week, on a mission to break from the juvenile rankings and into the senior rankings.

YOUTHFUL DEATH

In my second year of college, I was starkly reminded about life's fragility and the certainty that none of us are getting out of this life alive. Premature death struck my community again, cruelly taking 19-year-old Roy Power. It was simply heartbreaking.

Roy was a talented footballer and a competitor throughout my teenage years. He played for and captained Waterford Crystal FC, the main obstacle that faced my Tramore team for cup and league success each year. Many a competitive and enjoyable battle were shared between us and our teams over the years. More than opponents, we became teammates and classmates in secondary school, sitting beside each other for two years of English class and sharing laughs in the classroom, hallways and on the playing fields of De La Salle.

I hadn't seen Roy in about a year, since I left for college. My last memory of Roy was joking with him as he minded his Debs date's glitzy handbag like a gent, doing some modelling work with it.

'Looking smashing as ever, Roy,' I winked.

'Ah stop it, Al,' he laughed back, taking the piss with a glamorous pose.

My dad and I were in Portugal, enjoying our first holiday away with just the two of us, when I got a missed call and then a text from my old football captain, telling me Roy had died. He had taken his own life. I went from having the time of my life with Dad to the harrowing news knocking me for six, jolting me out of my privileged, happy bubble. It was a bewildering and horrifying thing to try to process, thinking of Roy experiencing such a rough patch of despondence, suffering to that extent and taking an irreversible course of action. The tragedy was such an upsetting waste of a young man's future, the bright light of his potential extinguished forever.

Suicide takes the lives of 800,000 people every year, according to the World Health Organisation. The trauma affects millions more: friends, families, and communities left reeling. That is a hell of a lot of people sharing similar difficulties. Sadly, it's something that has affected my own family too; I had an uncle, Seamus, take his life before I ever got to know him.

While experiencing low points as everyone does, self-harm and suicide have not been considerations I've personally had to grapple with. I can't for a minute imagine what it must feel like to struggle with those dark thoughts. I'd plead with anyone struggling to cope, to seek assistance and communicate their thoughts and feelings with their GP, the Samaritans, counsellors or loved ones. We should view our mind as we would any other body part and get advice and treatment when we realise something isn't quite right. These drastic moments are preventable.

It was yet another painful and unwelcomed reminder to live with intent and purpose. I felt I needed to pay more attention to what truly mattered, and make sure I was grateful for the health and opportunities afforded to me, and to try to lead a full life to the best of my ability.

ADJUST AND TRY AGAIN

After an unsuccessful year on the track, I decided to make a change and switch up my training group. I switched to Clonliffe Harriers coaching guru, John Shields, out in Santry, north Dublin. This was another high-level group of track athletes, including Brian Gregan, who can run a blistering 45-second 400-metre lap time. My old Ferrybank training partners, competitors and friends Gavin Kennedy and Chris Russell, were there too. I felt right at home from the word go.

The new training commute, from Phibsborough to Santry, wasn't too much better than that from Rialto to Ringsend in first year. I'd head off for training around 05:00 p.m., leaving Robbie and Barry, my housemates, to carry on enjoying their season of FIFA, having a few cheap cans and possibly enjoying a joint. I'd leave about an hour to get to the track, a longish walk past Mountjoy Prison to make it to the unpredictable bus, before standing in the city's evening traffic. I'd spend an hour and a half training on the track and about another hour to get home to the lads, who'd still be enjoying their evening of PlayStation or getting ready for a night on the town. We lived together but worlds apart in many ways.

The primary motivation for switching my training group was because their schedule enabled me to venture home to Waterford on weekends. I missed my friends and family and had a girlfriend, Laura, who I had become increasingly attached to over the summer. I got Clonliffe Harriers' core track sessions in mid-week in Dublin. Instead of doing Clonliffe's session on the weekend, I hopped into Ferrybank AC's similar Saturday morning session, trying to stick with my clubmate Thomas Barr.

Being away from Ferrybank AC for a year, I felt I was going backwards on my return to these weekend hill sprints at home. I was used to whooping Thomas over the years, on our staple session of 3 x 180 metres, 180 metres, 120 metres. He was younger and was more of a high jumper than a sprinter. He was not only keeping up with me now but was getting further ahead of me the deeper into the rounds we charged. It made me doubt myself, big time. I didn't know at the time – nobody did – but Thomas was whacking up the dial, steadily turning himself into an elite Irish sprint legend. He'd later finish fourth in the Rio 2016 Olympic 400-metre hurdles final, earn a bronze medal at the 2018 European Athletics Championships and capture the Irish National Record (48.65 seconds). It gives me goosebumps and a huge smile reading and writing about my friend's incredible achievements. At least hindsight has made these training-session beat downs by the young gun – puking up while trying to keep up – much more bearable for me to come to terms with.

The switch in training group certainly made my life more enjoyable, not spending long weekends alone anymore. The effort remained constant and training continued five, six, seven times per week, hitting the track, the hills and the road. I was upping efforts in the weights room too, under the guidance of Jim Kidd's son, Andy Kidd.

After another year of putting the work in, I'd expected to see the fruits of my labour on the track come race time. Just in time for the competition season, I acquired an overuse injury. Training in discomfort for weeks, the unpleasant feeling in my foot wasn't going away. When the discomfort turned to pain, I went to the physio who recommended I get an MRI scan. The scan found that I had a stress fracture in a bone on the top of my foot. The repeated impact of my foot against the unforgiving track, jumping over hurdles and snapping it back to earth as quickly as I could, caused the bone's outside layer to weaken and crack gradually. Under doctor's orders, any hope of a race season was down the swanny before it even got going. All the hours of hard work and sacrifice throughout the year were for nothing.

I was at my wits' end with the sport at this point. Rather than focus on the negative frustration I could do nothing about, I looked to the silver lining. I couldn't train or race for the summer season, so I focused on just enjoying being a teenager for those months, spending more time with my girlfriend, going to pubs and clubs and a festival, without the demanding training and competition schedule preventing it.

QUIT!

I know all the motivational posters and videos in the world say that you should never give up – don't quit. In my opinion, that's a load of bollocks! After spending a decade of sprint training, making the sacrifices to have a stab at the transition to senior level in college, I decided it was time for me to call it a day. There was little to no pleasure in the hours spent commuting alone, to push to, and through, intense discomfort, just to clock mediocre times or not race at all in the end. The effort was simply not worth the reward anymore. I felt like I would be flogging a dead horse if I continued to compete, as my heart was no longer in it.

The first two years of college, aged 17-19, were pivotal in finding out if I could hack it as a senior athlete. My times weren't improving despite the effort over that critical period. I wasn't going to make the grade. I also knew that sprinting was way too taxing to be a casual hobby. I didn't know what was next for me, but I knew sprinting wasn't it.

I'm an advocate for trying, trying and trying again. Still, if something's consistently not working out, dragging you down, rather than lifting you, despite trying different angles and making best endeavours, then I say quit! Refocus the time and energy towards other aspects of your life, or create and develop new elements to your existence.

Despite the simplistic motivational talk, I think quitting can often be a catalyst for personal growth, improved wellbeing and increased enjoyment of life. Imagine if you reached a pay, title, knowledge or responsibility ceiling in a workplace at the age of 25. Never quit? Don't give up? No! The blanket application of inspirational clichés just doesn't hold weight in reality. If I believed I could learn, grow, be more valued and happier elsewhere, quitting is *probably* the best call in that scenario.

I say *not quitting* can be harmful, like staying in an abusive relationship, a miserable job, or sinking all your time and money into the same *repeatedly* failing venture, at the expense of family, friends and wellbeing. I emphasised *repeatedly* in case people think I'm giving people a pass when they give up after dipping their toe in the icy water, declaring they tried to swim but found it too challenging, or didn't enjoy it. Quit, yes – but for your own sake, don't wuss out before a proper immersion!

In my case, I knew that after putting in years and years of graft, I'd reached a ceiling that I couldn't push through, despite the different lines of attack, with Ferrybank AC, DSD AC and Clonliffe Harriers AC. My full honest effort enabled me to confidently look myself in the mirror, satisfied in the knowledge that I gave it my best shot and wasn't good enough. I felt zero shame or embarrassment in the ultimate outcome as those feelings are attached to not trying at all or not trying my best in the given circumstance. It would have been an entirely different kettle of fish if I'd prematurely made the decision before my move to Dublin and went straight from the juvenile ranks to a bar stool. In that scenario, I would have always looked back in regret and thought *I had potential! What if ...?*

Knowing when to call it a day is something we all must accept at some point. Sprinting defined me up until that point. Closing the door on my comfort zone and walking into the unknown was scary and intimidating. After debating with myself, I viewed it as an opportunity. By quitting, I had created 15 more hours a week to do as I chose. There was an exciting sense of freedom created by my decision.

Shortly after deciding to quit athletics, my 18-month relationship ended with an emotional mess. It was a monumental adjustment in such a short space of time for a young fella to deal with. With my regimented athletics lifestyle off the table and serious girlfriend gone, there was a vast blank canvas in front of me. The heartbreak and the openness and uncertainty of the road ahead were overwhelming. *Where do I go from here? What am I going to do now?*

I took a walk by myself to clear my head from the anger, sadness, and confusion and somehow came up with the notion of running around Ireland – no rhyme nor reason! Admittedly, my head was all over the place as the idea popped out of nowhere, but it had an adventurous, romantic ring to it and struck a chord at the time. In hindsight, it's a funny memory – a sulking teenager moping around the housing estate block, trying to get over a girl and dreaming up adventures as a coping mechanism. While Sinead O'Connor was sullenly musing in my earphones about being able to eat her dinner in a fancy restaurant and sleep with whoever she chose, I was there thinking *I'm my own man now, and I can run anywhere I feckin' want.* I probably won't make it as a songwriter, to be fair.

As part of those stable and rational teen breakup brainwaves I was getting, and in light of no longer having the training and competition regiment, I decided to swim with the tide and embrace change. That chaotic summer, I researched the Erasmus Programme, an EU initiative that encourages students to do part of their third level education abroad. The DIT Town Planning Department only had one established Erasmus link, with a German university, but I hadn't a word of German. Instead, I decided to try to blaze my own trail. Somehow, I landed on the University of Dundee. I went about establishing a new link, liaising with both colleges to try to get an agreement.

I was successful with the initiative and was the first DIT Town Planner to go there. I realise Ireland and Scotland are not exactly the contrasting cultures the exchange initiative was established to foster, but I couldn't have cared less. My parents would benefit from an EU Erasmus grant, awarded to students for partaking in the programme, and would save a bomb not having to pay Dublin rent costs. I was going to get to feck off on an adventure somewhere new and have something to distinguish my CV from the other Irish graduates, which I thought sensible in a time of recession and poor job prospects. It felt like perfect timing to create an experience to look forward to for the second half of my third year at college.

THREE LITTLE BIRDS

Before I got to Scotland, lightning struck once again when my friend, Gary O'Keefe, died tragically in September 2010. It took the air from my lungs and words from my mouth. We had been out at a few sessions over the previous couple of weeks, having right craic together. I couldn't believe it. Gar was a healthy 21-year-old surfing enthusiast. *How could this be happening again?* The shock of death wasn't any easier to process.

Gary had just returned to Dublin for the first week of the college term, went to bed and didn't wake up. It was a case of Sudden Cardiac Death. It was heart-rending for everyone, made more poignant as it couldn't have happened to a nicer fella and family. I don't recall any interaction with Gary ending without having a smile, or a laugh, or feeling better for the exchange. The community were in shock at yet another tragic loss of young life.

Gary's laid-back nature and good vibes were epitomised by the song chosen to lead his coffin out of the church, Bob Marley's 'Three Little Birds'. The Jamaican drums blasted the distinctive tune:

'Don't worry, about a thing, 'cause every little thing gonna be all right.'

There was a mixture of smiles, laughter and sobbing, knowing he would have appreciated the anthem blaring around the church, the music encouraging people to reminisce on the good times shared.

I know I have discussed death quite a bit, but the prevalence of premature death in my life has had a profound impact on me. The unexpected deaths of Nicole, Roy and Gary have shaped my attitude and thought process. These times of sorrow flipped everything and forced me into a truer perspective, appreciating the finite nature of it all. In those awful times, there is clarity on what has value and what does not. I often remind myself how fortunate I am to be breathing today, with an acute awareness of the precarious nature of life.

Confucius is reputed to have said, 'We have two lives, and the second begins when we realise we only have one.' I feel a duty to live to the full because that opportunity doesn't exist for all those young friends. I need to prove myself worthy of this opportunity and not squander it. Those that were lost are never too far from my thoughts.

TERRY FOX

I left home for Scotland in January 2011. This opportunity

contributed substantially to my lap of Ireland challenge. In fact, if I hadn't gone to Scotland, it's likely I would not have embarked on the charity challenge at all – or written this book. Without the strict regimen of five to seven training sessions per week, I had more time than I knew what to do with. Lecturing hours were way less demanding in Scotland too: a handy eight hours of lectures a week. It was the most alone I'd been, so I quickly set about making friends. I got a job doing nightclub promotions and joined the GAA club for training – well, I went to one training session and then joined the parties.

On one of my first nights in Dundee I made friends with a great bunch of Americans and Canadians at the international student's welcome night. There were about 30 people at the pub, gulping their drinks and doing their best to survive the initial awkwardness of the newbie's networking event.

The Scottish student volunteer welcomed everyone and said, 'I think it would be a good place to start if we say what our names are, where we're from and what we're studying, so we can all get a sense of the international spread in the room.'

'I'm from Toronto, Canada.'

'I'm from North Carolina, USA.'

'I'm from Tasmania, Australia.'

I looked up from my pint of Guinness and realised it was my turn. Trying to hold a straight face, I announced my back story with a thick Irish accent. The room of real foreign exchange students erupted with laughter.

'Sláinte,' I raised my glass, laughing back.

A few weeks later, I got chatting to one of the Canadians,

Stephen Lavender.

'Oh, you're a runner, eh? What do you make of Terry Fox then?' Stephen asked.

'I haven't clue who that is, sorry.'

'What? Seriously? He's only the baddest runner there is. He's a Canadian hero. You have to check him out on YouTube when you get a chance.'

Intrigued, I looked up Terry Fox. For those that don't know the story, I too suggest watching one of the short clips online. Terry attempted to run across Canada on what he called 'The Marathon of Hope', in 1980. He did this to raise money for cancer research. Like many kids, Terry was an avid sports participant growing up, which I related to. What was so mind-blowing, upsetting and inspirational about Terry was that he was dealt an awful hand in his teenage years. At the age of 18, Terry was diagnosed with bone cancer in his knee, forcing him to have his leg amputated above the joint. He didn't take the hardship lying down and set himself the seemingly impossible task of crossing Canada on one real foot and a prosthetic leg. He began this mammoth adventure, aged 21, after 14 months of training on the new prosthesis. As the saying goes, 'it's not what happens to you, but how you react to it that matters.' This guy epitomised that spirit.

I watched the YouTube video, welling up, as Terry hopped towards his goal. He talked about his cancer, the suffering he went through in chemotherapy, and the good he wanted to try to create out of the shitty hand life had dealt him. He recalled the horror of seeing people much younger than him in the cancer ward, mere children. Terry experienced people in his hospital ward dying around him, and it had a profound impact on his life's trajectory. He had to try to do something to help the situation, instead of sitting by on the sidelines as another victim of the cruel disease.

After 143 days and an incredible 5,373 kilometres, cancer had spread to his lungs, forcing Terry to stop his running dream. My heart was bleeding for this hero of a young fella. He died shortly after leaving his road run, on the 28th June 1981, at the age of just 22. His story and efforts struck a chord with me. I was in bits watching. It clearly hit home with others too. His hard work and self-sacrifice were not in vain, raising over $27,000,000 CAD for charity. The Terry Fox Foundation has since raised $800,000,000 CAD for cancer research! I was thinking, *How on earth have I not heard of this guy until now? This achievement is unbelievable!*

Terry's story inspired me. The short video made me feel like a right lazy git. I thought I wasn't contributing enough by merely studying for my undergraduate degree. I had more free time on my hands than ever before but was arguably wasting it, drinking, socialising and then trying to cure the hangover. Don't get me wrong: I enjoyed being a regular student for a change, slugging away at cheap spirits, but the novelty wore off and my lifestyle lacked any great meaning. Terry's video refocused my mind. *Will I ever be as time and health rich as now? Can I use the gift of time and health more effectively to better myself and effect even the smallest of positive changes?*

I was reminded of Eddie Izzard's running accomplishments too, and my hormone fuelled fantasy about running a lap of Ireland. The memory of deceased friends flooded back, with the associated feeling of urgency and responsibility to do better. It all suddenly seemed more tangible and a viable possibility for me. Maybe I just had too much time on my hands without training commitments and with the reduced lecture time, but ultra-distance running was now gaining more traction in my mind as each day passed.

An idea is one thing. Anyone can have an idea. Action is what separates the boys from the men. I didn't commit to a single thing or write it down anywhere. I certainly didn't mention this madcap idea to anyone either. I was spending more and more time going back and forth in my head, humming and hawing, trying to weigh up the pros and cons of trying to run around Ireland. *You could raise loads of money for good causes. You could fail miserably and look like an absolute plonker for thinking you could accomplish such a feat. You'd learn a new skill of endurance running. You could badly injure yourself. It would be an adventure, and you'd get to see new places. You've just got your time back to be normal; do you really want to give it all up again for training?* Once alone in the solitude of my room, on and on the indecisive internal dialogues went.

After a week or two, the idea was slowly consuming me, but I was still too hesitant. It was like the moment before jumping into the cold Irish sea from a height. It was a great idea in principle. I had driven there, got changed into my togs and was standing on the pier edge, but just as I coiled myself back to jump, I'd chicken out. I didn't have the guts. *This is an awful idea!* I lacked a kick up the arse to get me off the safe shore and into the deep cold waters; however, life would interject and settle the internal debate as the wheels flew off.

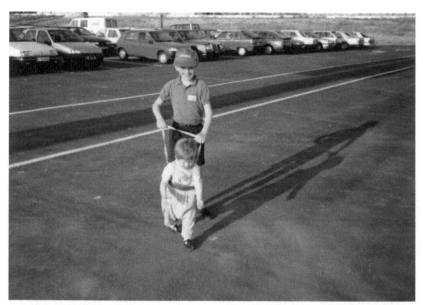

Being restrained by my big brother, Evan, since I was a liability if unsupervised.

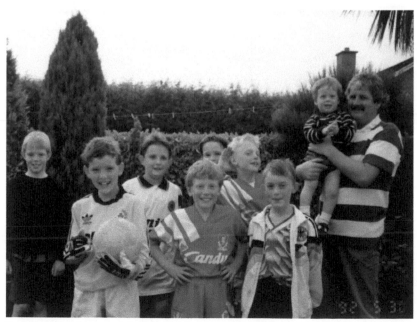

Dad looking after me while the big boys played at my brother's 10th birthday party.

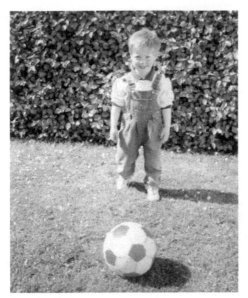

Starting them young.

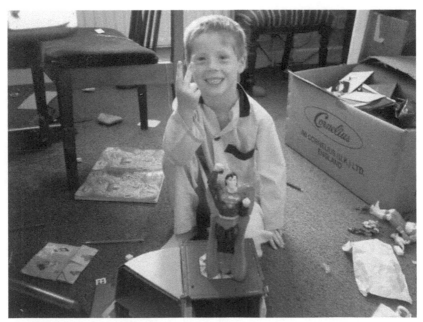

'Do the Superman pose, Alan'.

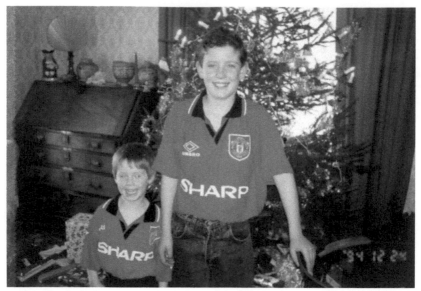

Christmas in Tramore, 1994, getting matching Man Utd jerseys with Evan.

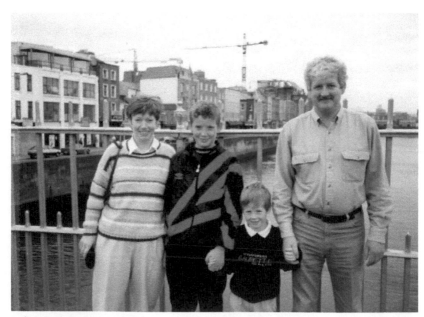

A family daytrip to Dublin with my mam, brother and dad.

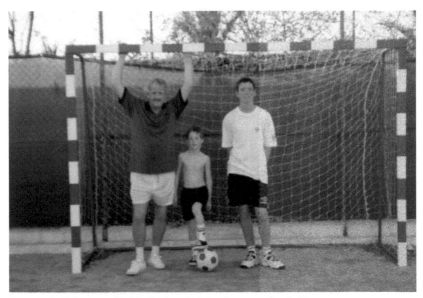

Even on holidays, we had to find a pitch to play some football.

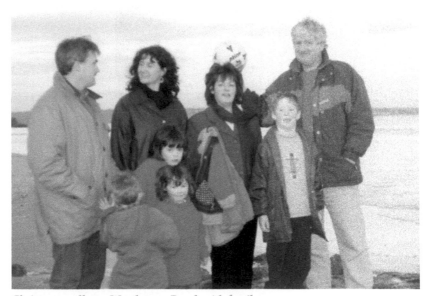

Christmas walks on Woodstown Beach with family.

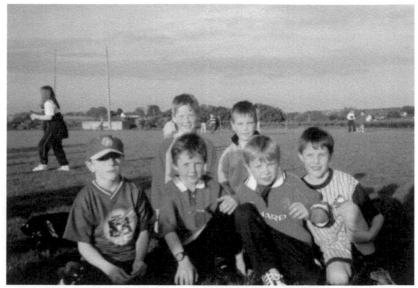

Ballygunner school sports day with my friends and classmates. Front, from left to right: Gavin Kennedy, Gary Murphy, Philip Mahony, David Redmond. Back, from left to right: Me and Robert Whelan.

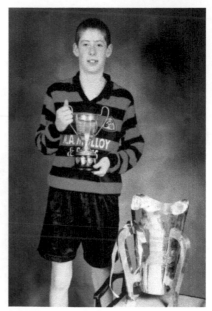

Winning some Gaelic Football trophies for Ballygunner Primary School.

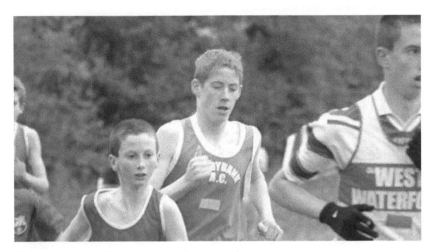

Waterford County Cross Country Championships.

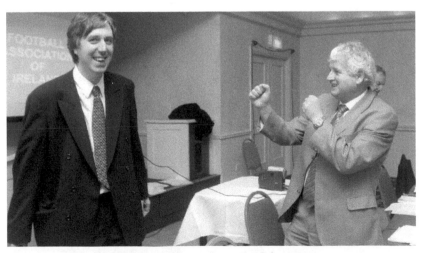

My dad enjoying his work for the Football Association of Ireland with John Delaney.

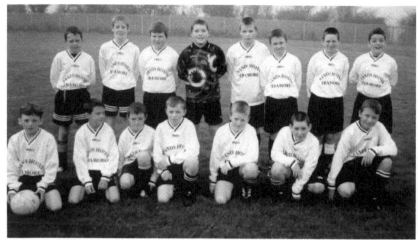

Tramore AFC, where I spent countless hours playing football. Back Row, from left to right: Alex Flynn, me, Darren O'Meara, Martin O'Neill, Trevor Douglas, Craig Lennon, Gavin Falconer, Sam Shanahan. Front row, from left to right: Zach Shanahan, Robbie Flynn, Robbie Palmer, Paul Farrelly, Ricky Hutchinson, Michael O'Sullivan, Niall Murphy.

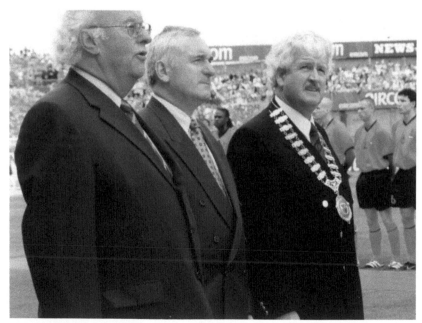

My dad doing his pre-match duties as the President of the Football Association of Ireland, in 2001, alongside the former Taoiseach, Bertie Ahern.

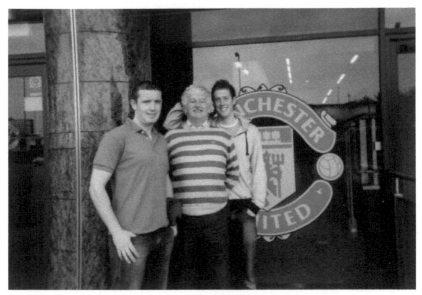

Messing about at Old Trafford with my brother and Dad.

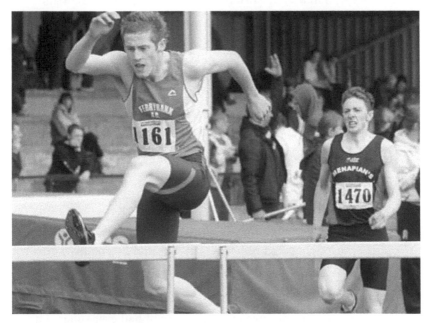

The last hurdle before winning the under-19 400 metre hurdles All-Ireland Championships, with my old classmate and clubmate, Gavin Kennedy, in a close second.

FOUR:

REALITY STRIKES

STROKE

On the 15th March 2011, halfway through my semester in Scotland, life hit me like a bus. I received a sombre call from my mam.

'Hi Al, all okay?'

'Yeah, great thanks, Mam.'

'Can you talk?'

'Yeah, sure. Just in my room. How're things?'

'Not too good today. I'm in the hospital with Dad. He's alright though, just in a bed and getting the treatment he needs. He's had a stroke.'

'Is he okay? Do I come home? What can I do?'

'No, no, you stay put. He'll recover; he just needs to rest up. They're looking after him well; I'm here and Ev's on his way.'

To be honest, the seriousness didn't register with me during the short call. I didn't know anything about strokes at the time. No friends, family, or anyone I was aware of had ever suffered a stroke. Mam was protecting me, downplaying the gravity of the situation, because there was nothing I could do from Scotland. She didn't want to panic or upset me, especially as it was the furthest I'd lived from home and my longest duration away from home too. Mam just let me know what happened, that Dad was stable and it would all be okay.

I immediately hopped onto Google and started learning. This was my first time finding my way to the Irish Heart Foundation's website. The not-for-profit organisation seemed the most reliable source of information. I quickly discovered that a stroke is a life-threatening condition that occurs when the blood supply to part of the brain is cut off[1]. Blood supply can be interrupted by a burst blood vessel, called a Haemorrhagic stroke, which accounts for about 15% of strokes. A blocked blood vessel causes the remaining 85% of strokes, and these are called Ischaemic strokes[2]. Damage to the brain can affect how your body works, and as scary as it is, it can also change how you think, feel and behave[3].

The term 'stroke' comes from the fact that it usually happens without warning, 'striking' the person down out of nowhere. I say 'usually', as people can sometimes suffer Transient Ischemic Attacks (TIA) in advance of a stroke. TIA's are also referred to as 'mini-strokes' or 'warning strokes'. Mini-strokes cause stroke-like symptoms that resolve within minutes, or 24 hours at the most, with the shorter, temporary blockage of blood supply, causing no permanent damage. However, more than a third of people who have a mini-stroke and don't get emergency treatment, have a full-blown stroke within one year. This 'mini' warning sign provides patients and doctors with a crucial window of opportunity for urgent medical intervention to prevent a future stroke[4].

The effects of a stroke on the body are immediate, and the sooner a person receives treatment for a stroke, the less damage is likely to happen. I hope, by now, people have seen the Irish Heart Foundation's 'Act F.A.S.T.' awareness campaign. This campaign was designed to help the public recognise when someone is suffering a stroke. It's essential to call 999 immediately if someone's face has fallen or drooped to one side, if they can't raise and keep both of their arms raised or if they're slurring their speech.

Stroke is the second leading cause of death worldwide, behind heart disease[5]. About 10,000 people in Ireland suffer a stroke each year, and around 2,000 die. This is more deaths than breast cancer, prostate cancer and bowel cancer combined[6], illustrating how severe and common a threat to life it is.

Approximately 100,000 people suffer a stroke each year in the UK. In England, Wales and Northern Ireland, the average age for someone to have a stroke is 74 for men and 80 for women, but strokes do not exclusively impact older people and can occur at any age, striking children and adults alike. Of those that survive the brain injury, many are never the same again. Survivors often have permanent disabilities. In fact, stroke is a leading cause of disability, with almost two-thirds of stroke survivors leaving the hospital with at least one form of disability. If someone is fortunate enough to survive having a stroke, they're far from in the clear. Stroke survivors have a 25% chance of having another stroke within five years of the initial one. The most significant cause for concern is within the first 30 days when the risk of a repeat stroke is at its highest[7]. These repeat strokes will hinder the difficult rehabilitation process at best and kill the person at worst.

You can imagine the disbelief and panic that was setting in as I read. I hadn't even got to the plethora of devasting effects of a stroke, including personality changes and problems with walking, speaking, understanding, reading, writing, swallowing, memory ... and on and on the eye-opening list went (see full details in Appendix 2).

Jesus Christ, I thought. I was reasonably calm after my mother's initial call: she'd done a great job reassuring me and shielding me from the gravity of the situation. But now I had equipped myself with some knowledge; the panic level shot straight to a 10 out of 10. I immediately picked up the phone.

'Mam, I just read up about strokes. He's far from being out of the woods. When's the soonest I can leave and get home? I should be there.'

'He has the doctors and nurses, and me and Ev are here to give a hand too. You'd be just standing around. There's really nothing extra that can be done. At least not now. We've discussed it and think it's best you prioritise passing your exams in May before coming home. Dad will be fine, and we'll look after him until you get home, okay? We can call and Skype until then, once he's able to.'

This was a bit of a white lie for my benefit. As I later discovered, at that stage Dad was incapacitated. He was unable to sit himself up in his hospital bed, never mind get out of it. Dad couldn't communicate effectively either, only able to slur a few swear words, in a state of complete frustration and confusion. He was fully with it, taking in and understanding what was going on around him, but couldn't do anything. With time and hindsight, Dad would later joke about the loss of language skills and swearing like Father Jack, but lying there only able to slur 'fuck' was no joke. It was traumatic for both him, experiencing the inability to communicate, and my family watching on helplessly by his side.

As useless as I probably would have been at home, I felt worthless, selfish and guilty for not being there with Dad, Mam and Ev. That's mostly what family is: just being there for each other, a crutch when it's needed.

With no means of my own to get home, and unwavering parental instruction to stay and pass my exams, I didn't have a choice in the matter.

My dad had only recently turned 60. In my youthful bliss, the mortality of my parents had never crossed my mind. Sure, I knew they would die, but I cushioned it with a lie. They'll be here for at least another 20 or 30 years, I'm certain. The reality was a difficult pill to swallow, made even more challenging by being geographically isolated. With the statistics I had read about stroke's common recurrence, I now didn't know if I'd see Dad alive again. If I did, what kind of person would be left to go home to when May came around? I was scared and could only imagine what Dad was going through.

The present was terrifying, and the uncertain future even more so. The main thing to focus on was that Dad had survived. Although in limbo, he could breathe, which gave us a glimmer of optimism that he would recover. We had to be grateful we were given that much, a luxury many stroke sufferers and their families aren't afforded. We latched onto the hope that Dad would muster all the resourcefulness and drive that we knew he possessed, to give himself the best chance at being one of the lucky ones. We'd tell ourselves that he's up for the fight – 'No better man for the job,' we'd say.

I think most of us are guilty of becoming comfortable in our routines, taking our day to day lives and health for granted. It can take moments of suffering to force us to open our eyes, appreciate what we have and pay attention. Dad's stroke lit a fire under me. Life's fragility hit me like a tonne of bricks once more. I cried myself to sleep but didn't want to talk about my family's struggle with anyone. I kept up lectures, the part-time job and the boozy nights out with new friends but, when the distractions stopped, alone, in the stillness of my dorm room, things were difficult. It didn't take me long to realise I was in deep shit emotionally and needed some tools to climb out.

I'm a simple, rational thinker. If something isn't right, I know it's not going to get any better by moaning or sitting on my arse, feeling sorry for myself. I had to be proactive and fight. Talking to others is strongly encouraged by professionals in moments like these and is one of the tools I recommended earlier. But, at this stage of my life, I didn't think talking was going to have any bearing on the root of the problem – my dad suffering a stroke and me not being there for my family at a critical time. I couldn't stop my dad having had the stroke, or stop him having another stroke for that matter, and I couldn't be there for another two months either.

I couldn't control these facts, so there was no point dwelling on them. Yet doing nothing created a feeling of complete inadequacy and uselessness. *What can I do to get through this moment?* I asked myself. I had to do something to make up for not being there or something that would make me feel like I was contributing in some way.

Dad's stroke changed everything. Whilst I had held myself back and couldn't convince myself to commit to my running dream during the previous month or two, my mindset changed. I needed to break out of the self-imposed confines of fear and switch from thinking what could go wrong, to focusing on what could go right. After his stroke, I reflected on a valuable lesson that Dad taught me as a child. When I was about 10 years old, he drove me on the back roads from home to Tramore, to play a football match. He must have noticed the hesitation in my previous games, which negatively impacted my performance and my team's performance.

'Listen, you can't be afraid to shoot. If you don't shoot, you'll never score. It's that simple. If the opportunity comes today, just give it a bash and have a shot. Worst case scenario: you'll miss, and you can try again, can't you? Or you'll set up a goal or score yourself. Just try.'

It's memorable because, with those words in the forefront of my mind that day, I took a punt and scored a screamer against Villa FC. I was miles outside the box, where no one was expecting it from. I even surprised myself with the shot at goal. Had Dad not encouraged me to take more risks that day, I wouldn't have shot from a silly distance in a million years and also wouldn't have scored the goal and won the game.

Sometimes our brains can overcomplicate the risk versus reward balancing act. The only way to guarantee failure is by not trying at all. When reality punched me in the face again, I realised I was being way too risk-averse and practical, instead of following my heart. I had *nothing* to lose in trying. I was a single, broke, 20-year-old student without responsibility, for god's sake – not a 40-year-old with underlying health conditions, a mortgage, a wife, and three children relying on my earnings to contribute to our survival. This was precisely the time in my life when I should be going out on a limb to do whatever took my fancy.

One thing was almost inevitable, if I didn't give the dream a bash, I'd likely still feel rudderless, and I'd forever regret not making the most of my time, youth and health. *You will achieve something positive in the effort*, I convinced myself. *Worst case, you'll get outside more, improve your health through high-quality leisure, pursue a passion and learn something new.* If that's what failure looked like, I could live with it.

Without any research, the decision was made. I was now a man with a mission, with a no retreat mindset. There were no longer any questions or doubt in my mind. This all-consuming sense of obligation got me out of the hole I'd found myself in and got me feeling useful, invigorated and alive. I was focused on hope, achieving something worthwhile with my life and overcoming life's adversity. Making the commitment to take meaningful action soothed the chaos and turmoil.

Until the third year of college, sport had always been my constant, an essential component in my upbringing, with short, medium and long-term goals. I had discarded it a few months prior but needed that support mechanism and structure more than ever. Turning to sport to express myself in this low point felt like the natural response.

As well as wanting to do it for my own sake, I desperately wanted to give my dad something to look forward to, something to get excited about again, a project I hoped we could work towards as a team. The challenge gave me a sense of optimism in a time of difficulty, and I wanted to try to extend that feeling to Dad. *Maybe this might give him more cause to fight.*

As well as the self-expression and self-development and family-centric reasons for pursuing the adventure, there was the ambition to do something which might contribute to the broader community, inspired by the phenomenal impact made by Terry Fox and Eddie Izzard. Trying to raise money for charity added an extra layer of responsibility, motivation and a sense of purpose related to my dad's stroke. It wasn't going to be just about me, or my family, but making a wider positive impact.

If I was a musician, I might have composed a song, or if I was an artist, I could have painted. I wasn't those things. I was a runner. Persistence and showing up was the skill I'd honed my entire life, and I'd try to use it to generate some good. With the Irish Heart Foundation leading the charge on stroke prevention and minimising the harmful impacts through the F.A.S.T. awareness campaign, they were a no brainer for me to dedicate my efforts to.

ADVANCING

With the decision made to start, I needed to decide when. 'Someday' isn't on the calendar, so I had to get specific and intentional, working towards a set deadline. I didn't know how long my dad had. That's always the case, but now I couldn't ignore this. I was afraid that he would suffer another stroke and that next time he wouldn't be so lucky. There was a sense of urgency in my project. The sooner I could do the challenge, the more likely Dad could be a part of it, and the more likely I could make him proud of my achievement.

Conversely, though, the less time I took to train and prepare, the less likely I was to succeed, and the less likely Dad could actively participate, as it would be too early in his recovery.

Summer 2011 was only a few weeks away. Eddie Izzard only did a few weeks of training before setting out on 43 marathons over 51 days. Although training didn't appeal to Eddie, the idea of walking injured, grunting and hobbling 10-plus hour marathons was much less appealing to me. I was a runner. I wanted to learn from Eddie's mistakes and be reasonably prepared to glide instead of plod. Terry Fox trained for 14 months to prepare for his 143-day running epic, in which he covered 5,373 kilometres. He had to get used to his prosthetic leg, too, mind you. The answer seemed to lie between four weeks and 14 months of training time with the answer likely closer to 10 months, given Terry's sizeable handicap.

Given that Dad couldn't even speak to me on the phone and the fact that there was enough stress on my family, my dad's rehabilitation had to be his primary focus. Dad couldn't get involved in my run if he wasn't better. That quickly ruled summer 2011 out for me. I wanted my family to be integral to the challenge, and I wanted to give a good account of myself and my family. I knew we needed more time.

Winter was about eight months out, but I'd have to start prepping immediately, as I was completely unprepared and clueless about where to even begin distance training. Dad was even less prepared to deal with the cards he had been dealt. It seemed unimaginable that he could recover in that short timeframe. I felt it was too close. Winter would be unnecessarily grim, too, in terms of weather and an insufficiently prepared body and mind. With the clock ticking in my head, I decided summer 2012, roughly one year away, was realistic for us both. I'd have time to sort the logistics, prepare my body and complete my final year at college. Dad would have time to do his best to try to drag himself out of the hospital and back to his feet.

Once the decision was made and I'd settled on a project timeline, I had to keep advancing with little steps. Although I was gung-ho for running a lap of Ireland, I had no idea what the distance was. If I had any sense, I probably would have thought about that before committing to my romantic notions! I did a rough Google Maps measurement, broadly joining the four corners of Ireland, including the main towns and cities on the route. I discovered it was around 1,500 kilometres. I divided the total distance by 42.2 kilometres (one marathon) and got 35 marathons. *That's certainly good to know,* I thought. Ignorance is bliss. I'd never even run a half-marathon, my longest run being 16 kilometres, so the task's scale didn't even register in the slightest.

I was naively unconcerned about the numbers before my eyes. One step at a time, *I'll be grand,* was my thinking, and it got me out of the starting blocks.

I had committed with a clear purpose, settled on a project timeline and broad route, and now knew the distance. I was taking vital baby steps. That's what this marathon journey required. Thinking of it as 10 million steps makes it unfathomable to conceive. The mind says, *that's too much. It's impossible.* I needed to trick my mind. *One step? I can do that for sure. How about one more now? That last step was okay. I think I can handle one more.* By focusing on the present action, we can end up halfway up the mountainside with a view behind us before realising our progress. When we've gone that far and can see the trail of work, continuing upwards seems logical, rather than retreating off the mountain having only gone halfway. People can get lost in the intimidating scale of successful mountain summits, fat-loss targets, or operating a successful business, but can forget these achievements must all start with the most modest and mundane initial steps. I had to establish my motivations for doing it, commit to myself, plan the multiple practical steps to get to the end goal and start patiently moving forward, trusting in the process.

THE MARATHON STUDENT

I'd assumed someone had run this route before and thought they'd be the key to helping me. I began my search online and discovered heaps of cyclists, some kayakers and even a lad that hitch-hiked around Ireland with a fridge. I couldn't find any runners completing a lap of the country, or even trying to. I'd assumed every type of physical feat of endurance had already been done at this stage. On the other hand, it was a fairly niche cup of tea, alright. *What kind of person would want to do that?* A naive student with no marathon experience – that's who! It certainly added a buzz, knowing I'd be the first to try and it gave me even more incentive to prove to myself that I can be the person who gets the job done.

Not a physical step was taken but steady progress nonetheless, learning that it was unprecedented. The run's total length was similar to what Eddie Izzard had completed and was less than what Terry Fox had done on a prosthetic limb, so that was some comfort. The 1,500-piece jigsaw had the corner pieces in place. These small wins were having a snowball effect, encouraging me to get more parts in place. The satisfaction and excitement created by my productivity were also distracting from my upset and concern about the situation at home. That was a welcome by-product.

As a challenge aimed at fundraising for charity, I didn't think the distance alone would be enough to capture the public's imagination – at least not to the extent that it would compel total strangers to part with their hard-earned cash. To make the endeavour more donation-worthy, I concluded that I needed to make it tougher and catchier. To stack the odds even further against me, I decided, in my foolishness, that running it as consecutive marathons was the only way to go! Oh, sweet summer child. What that meant was completing 35 marathons in 35 consecutive days.

I thought it had a nice ring to it. It seemed a much easier

sell than, say, 35 marathons with one day's rest per week. I didn't give it a second thought. I wouldn't be scheduling days off to try to allow my body to rest up from the toll of the previous days. The damage would be accumulated, and I would likely be broken, but this added a twisted appeal to the challenge. *Will I be able to suck it all up, tough it out and keep going? Only one way to find out!*

Although I had spent almost a decade sprint training, I had never joined the distance runners for a single training session. I hadn't the foggiest about marathon and ultra running and needed to become a devoted student of the discipline. With the challenge refined and arbitrary terms and conditions imposed, I decided it would be wise to seek help from people who have experience doing what I was aiming to do – or at least something similar.

Trawling online, I came across Dean Karnazes, an American full-time ultra-distance runner. In 2006, sponsored by The North Face, he ran 50 marathons in 50 states in 50 days. The images looked phenomenal: a huge branded tour bus and support jeep, branded inflatable finish archway and street stalls, crowds of participants and supporters, as well as a ginormous team of professionals keeping the tour on the road and making sure each day's event ran smoothly. The scale of his no-expense-spared operation made my eyes open wide. I began feeling more out of my depth, reading the guy's credentials. Before Dean's back-to-back marathon challenge, he had run 560 kilometres in 81 hours straight. He was also the winner of the Badwater Ultramarathon (217 kilometres), a notorious race across Death Valley, in 50°C temperatures. I can't even sit in that sort of climate, never mind walk or run in it. He seemed superhuman. Even with that experience, he still put in 15 months of targeted training for his 50/50/50 event. During the challenge itself, he typically ran each of the marathons in between three-and-a-half and four-and-a-half hours. *Fuckin' hell*, I thought. There was no comparison between him and me – the lowly inexperienced student.

Dean Karnazes was Manchester United, and I was the local team of weekend warriors. I admired him but avoided the comparison trap. I had no aspirations to put on such a mammoth event with 50 mass participation races and 50 expos. Although not competing with Dean or comparing myself to him, there was definitely a lot I could learn from him. I ordered all his books and sent him an email straight away, crossing my fingers that he'd respond. Given the man's training, racing, speaking and TV commitments, it was no surprise that I didn't hear back from Dean at the time, but his books gave me invaluable insights. I was never a book worm – I hadn't the time with school and sports. Still, I enjoyed this learning process, absorbing as much information as possible, actively taking notes and underlining what might be useful for the months ahead.

My online investigation threw up a much more accessible and relatable ultra-distance runner: Gerry Duffy from Mullingar. Gerry and his friend Ken Whitelaw had also read of Dean Karnazes' exploits and were inspired to try to replicate them, Irish style. They completed 32 marathons in 32 counties in 32 days, in 2010. They raised an astonishing €500,000 for charity, with some promotional help from Ryanair Chief Executive, Michael O'Leary.

I read that Gerry was in his forties and had been four stone overweight and a chain smoker, which gave me some reassurance and confidence back. Gerry seemed more of an Eddie Izzard type, plodding on, despite his excess weight and disadvantaged lungs. Given my youth and prime physical health, I thought, *I should at least be able to replicate that fella's efforts.* I should have dug a bit deeper in my research. At the time, I had failed to grasp that by 2010 Gerry was no longer a hefty 17-stone chain smoker, having long kicked the bad habits. He had completed multiple marathons, triathlons, Ironman triathlons, and even a double Ironman triathlon in the meantime. I was better off not knowing all that at the time, as it certainly would have brought my ability in to doubt again.

I dropped Gerry an email and waited in hope for some help. To my delight, Gerry actually responded. *Finally, a positive lead. Now we're sucking diesel!* What I badly needed was his training plan. *If it worked for him,* I thought, *it would surely work for me.* He didn't want to share his plan willy-nilly with some stranger online. However, he did offer to meet me in person instead. I guess he wanted to see if I was genuine, committed and deserving of his time and help. *Completely fair,* I thought. *He doesn't want to help timewasters.* By hook or by crook, I would get to him and show him I couldn't be any more serious about following through on my plans.

AFTERMATH

May arrived in no time. I sat my exams in Dundee and returned home from Scotland, not knowing what to expect when I saw my dad again. It was about two months since he had suffered the stroke at this stage. Dad was moved from Waterford Regional Hospital, where he had arrived with little to no speech or movement, to St Patrick's Hospital, Waterford, where he began his initial rehabilitation. Fortunately, he got a place in the National Rehabilitation Hospital (NRH) in Dún Laoghaire, without months of despair on a waiting list.

The NRH offers the most comprehensive range of specialist rehabilitation services in the country. It was a facility we were all so grateful for, especially Dad. He was given a regimented daily schedule at the start of each week and would get to work. He might have speech and language therapy first thing, then onto occupational therapy, physiotherapy, and then dietitian meetings, for example. He loved the structure and daily hard graft. Anything was better than lying in a hospital bed or getting sporadic treatment, with consequent slow progress. We shared his frustration when he was sitting there wallowing, feeling useless, but once there was a plan of action to follow, it lifted and focused all our hearts and minds.

By the time I got home to Waterford, my father was allowed home from the NRH for weekends. I didn't know what to say when I saw him. He was sitting in the living room with a walking frame next to him, waiting to see me. As I walked into the room, I could immediately see the toll his ordeal had taken on him. He wasn't able to stand up for our usual embrace. He appeared gaunt, his clothes loose, and his speech laboured and unclear. He was smiling, though. I was just delighted to be home and relieved to see Dad home too – down but by no means out. He was happy to see his family together again, in the comfort of our home.

Given his condition in the immediate aftermath of the stroke a few weeks earlier, I found it incredible that he was home so soon. Not only home, but shuffling about the house himself, albeit slowly and relying on the metal frame for support. As fast and as well as his symptoms were improving, Dad hated having lost his independence. I could see the fire and impatience in his eyes, wanting his freedom back. His attitude reassured me that he was going to give it all he had. Dad was determined to get back to himself as quickly as he could.

The specialists at the NRH had advised him to set himself goals as part of the rehabilitation process. Creating a target for him was part of my thinking when deciding to pursue the lap of Ireland run. I think the NRH and I both failed to factor in Dad's ambition and doggedness. He didn't need any encouragement. You thought I was unwise planning to run a lap of Ireland? Well, his targets were being able to drive again and taking a plane to London to watch Manchester United vs Barcelona, at Wembley Stadium, for the Champions League Final. He told the doctors about the medium to long-term driving ambition, alright. That would satisfy them that he was on the right path, setting ambitious yet realistic aims for some time down the road. He had more sense than to mention his Wembley ambition, for the obvious reason that it was only a few weeks away, on the 28th May. The game was a mere two months after his stroke. He knew they'd never sanction something like that so soon. He kept it a secret. On this occasion, he thought it better to ask for forgiveness than for permission.

One weekend morning, when it was just him and me at

home, I heard Dad blowing a fuse. I ran to the commotion, not knowing what to expect. I sighed with relief, finding him infuriated by the Ryanair website on his laptop, offering everything under the sun, but the flight.

'I want a flight to London,' the customer would tell the website.

'Would you like travel insurance?'

'No, just the flight.'

'Are you sure you don't want travel insurance? What about a car rental?'

'No, just the flight.'

'What about a hotel, and this or that?'

It was testing for the most zen person, never mind someone who had just suffered a brain injury, with the associated difficulty in controlling their emotions. It was a bit too much for him to handle at the time. I wanted to help, so asked what he was trying to do. He confided in me about the game and his plans to travel.

'Have the doctors cleared it? Never mind the doctors, what did Mam say about all this?'

'No, they don't know. I didn't ask. Are you going to help me or not?'

Whether I helped him or not, I knew he'd find a way. I wasn't going to tell him he couldn't do something that would be enjoyable, an achievement, something that would make him feel alive. Although it was probably ill-advised on medical grounds and premature in his recovery process, I supported his plan.

'You go out to the garden and try to breathe. I'll try to sort your flights out.'

I was left cursing at the website too but managed to book him his return tickets.

A fortnight later, the NRH staff waved him off for a weekend at home in Waterford, or so they thought. Like a mischievous child, he snuck off to the airport with his walking frame in tow and a friend by his side to chaperone.

Thankfully the trip went without any glitches. All's well that ends well. We pissed ourselves laughing when Dad recounted eventually telling the trusting NRH staff.

'Right, Milo, today I've set up some stairs for you. It's going to be a challenge so take your time. Would you like to try it? Think you'll manage?'

'I was up the steps in Wembley two weeks ago at the Champions League Final. I'm sure I can give it a go.'

Dad had to stop about three times with the laughter and amusement before being able to tell us about the short interaction. I could only imagine the brazen joy on his face telling the physical therapist – who, no doubt, had a look of utter disbelief. It's a priceless story that makes me smile every time. I guess it's safe to say I didn't lick it off the stones. I respected the risk he took to get to the match. He knew more than most that time is of the essence and he wanted to enjoy being part of the Champions League Final. It may seem reckless to some, but the risk of dying or having complications was worth the reward of living. He was pushing himself so that he could do the things he enjoyed doing in life, not so he could wrap himself in cotton wool for the rest of his days. It inspired me to plough on with my plans to ultra run first, before crawling or walking.

With his personal goal of attending the Champions League Final out of the way, it spurred Dad on towards his next mission: to learn to drive again. Driving was hugely important for him. Relying on others for getting him a beloved fresh blaa (a bread bun speciality of Waterford) or the newspaper depressed him no end. He was used to driving all over the country for matches and football meetings. Now he couldn't do it; it made him mad. Again, wanting to jump the gun and practise before the NRH would sanction him driving, he told me he was getting in his beloved car. I felt what a protective parent must feel about a child. I tried to reason that it was safer to wait for the docs to give the all-clear and drive in the controlled NRH centre. He felt he was ready now. My dad risked his life teaching me how to drive around car parks before being of age, so I thought it only fair that I supported him and returned the favour. We crawled around the housing estate in second gear for a bit, making sure to get the car back safely in position before Mam would find out and kill us for taking unnecessary risks. Doing something like that was so rewarding for him and built his confidence. It was also fiercely rewarding for me, being able to support him.

THE KEY

The primary weapon I knew I needed to reach the finish line of my 1,500-kilometre run was a training plan. If I couldn't find a hotel sponsor or afford it, I could stay in a tent or the back of a car. If I couldn't find a sponsor support vehicle or volunteers, I'd have to try to push my supplies in a buggy or hope I could rely on the use of the family car. If I couldn't find volunteer physios or have the funds to pay them, I'd have to make do with ice baths or bins, foam rolling and stretching. There were suboptimal workarounds for most things, but I didn't want a workaround for hours and hours of structured training. Although hugely time-consuming, training would make the ultimate challenge as enjoyable as possible compared to the excruciating untrained alternative. Gerry Duffy had the vital plan, and I just needed to get it.

Gerry Duffy was a busy man in May and June. He was finishing off his preparations for, and then competing in, a Deca Ironman race.

An Ironman triathlon consists of a 3.9-kilometre swim, a 180-kilometre cycle and a 42.2-kilometre marathon run. He was feckin' doing 10 of these … in 10 consecutive days! To his credit, he won the thing and was one of only three from the starting 20 to finish. In July, his schedule was chock-a-block too, launching his book, *Who Dares, Runs: The Remarkable Story of a Man who Went from 50 Lbs Overweight to Running 32 Marathons in 32 Consecutive Days*. Once I discovered this, I immediately bought it as another study aid. He was generous enough to offer his time in August to advise a kid with no experience and a wacky aspiration.

I was the beggar in this scenario, and we all know beggars can't be choosers. It was up to him to name the time and place, and I would say 'Perfect, thank you!' wherever or whenever that was. There's a big difference between having a goal and having a goal with a plan to achieve it. I knew the importance of the meeting with Gerry and, although it wasn't an easy place or time to make, I had to find a way.

Gerry was living in Mullingar and I was in Waterford.

I had no car, and he wanted to meet at 11:00 a.m. I was double jobbing it, working seven days a week over the summer holidays, scrubbing pots and pans in the Woodlands Hotel and being an unpaid intern in the Town Planning Department of Waterford County Council.

Clodagh, the hotel's head chef, knew I got on with my unpleasant job diligently. In the corner of the kitchen, I was in an old tracksuit, getting blasted by steam from the industrial dishwasher. Sweat soaked, my pink marigold rubber gloves and football jersey covered in leftover food, I was doing the minimum wage job nobody wanted to do and did it with a smile. Because of my enthusiastic approach to the menial tasks, Clodagh was more than happy to oblige my rare request for a shift change. Now I just needed to figure out how to get to Mullingar in time.

To make sure I made the meeting, I had to get up for 04:00 a.m. to get a 05:00 a.m. bus to Dublin. From Dublin, I'd need to wait for the connecting bus to Mullingar. There would be a six-hour journey for a one-hour meeting, followed immediately by a six-hour return journey. An essential 13 hours of effort to make the challenge possible.

The main hurdle to overcome wasn't getting time off work or getting to and from Mullingar, but the next stage of commitment: I would have to tell my parents. There was no way in hell I could leave the house at 04:00 a.m., returning 13 hours later, and not get the interrogation of a lifetime. I couldn't sneak it and would just have to come clean. I hadn't said a word about this ambition to anyone other than Dean Karnazes and Gerry Duffy. I respected these men, but they were strangers, so I didn't care if they thought I was a quitter or bullshitter. I knew once I told my parents it was a whole other ballgame. By saying the words aloud to my family, I would be setting expectations of the people closest to me. That's when things become real. It was a massive step for me as it sealed off the avenue of retreat.

I had to decide who to tell first, my mam or my dad. I'm not sure if it's the same in every household, but my mam is one of the most risk-averse people I know. She would wrap her sons in bubble wrap and put us in a safe if she could. I knew if I told her, she would think of all the things which could go wrong and the potential harm that could come to her baby. I knew she would suggest going back to track and field instead. That wasn't an option for me since it no longer contributed to my happiness and I didn't think sprinting 35 laps of the track in 35 days would inspire anyone to donate. Still, I could hear her voice of reason in advance of any conversation. Rather than worry Mam about it, I thought it best to confide in Dad first. This craic was much more up his alley. I knew he'd done some road running back in the day, so it wouldn't be entirely alien to him.

I invited my father out for breakfast the weekend before the planned trek to meet with Gerry. He knew something was up when I excluded Mam from the invite. On the drive to The Vee in Tramore, I remember feeling butterflies in my stomach. I had never felt nervous talking to Dad about anything, so it was an unusual feeling. Would he think I was an idiot for coming up with this? Or even more of an idiot for believing I could complete it? And more of an idiot yet again, to think I could do it with less than a year to prepare? Might he try to discourage me? What if he thought the health risks of putting my body under such extreme stresses were too much? Would I have two parents fixated on the potential damage I could cause myself or believing I was setting myself up to fail big time?

All these 'what if's' were racing around in my head.

We had our lovely breakfast, shooting the breeze and enjoying each other's company. When the post-breakfast teas came out, it was now or never.

'Right, I've got something to tell ya.'

'Okay. Spill the beans.'

I whipped out my giant Collins road map of Ireland. It nearly covered the breakfasts of the couple next to us. I could see his bewildered face, wondering, *where the feck is he going with this at all, at all?* I had marked Xs approximately every 42.2 kilometres, joined up, forming a continuous line around Ireland. He looked at the map with a smile and back to me.

'What's all this then?'

I was quite enjoying the dramatic unveiling at this stage and seeing his reaction.

'I'm going to run around that next summer for charity. Would you be up for helping me?'

He let out a little bemused laugh and a smile. I left him speechless for a tick, struggling to get the words outs. That might have been an effect from the stroke, controlling emotions, his breath and speaking – or it might have been a perfectly normal reaction.

'That's a hell of a distance,' he laughed in surprise.

I don't think he could have expected me to table this little venture, but he looked like he loved the idea.

'I've done a bit of homework. Two Irishmen recently did something similar, while a one-legged cancer patient did a comparable run in Canada. A professional runner did 50 marathons in 50 days in 50 states of the U.S, and a comedian did roughly the same craic in the UK. I think I can do it. I want the money raised to go towards the Irish Heart Foundation's Act F.A.S.T. stroke awareness campaign, and I'd like to donate a portion to your Football Village of Hope too.'

It gave him great joy to be involved in the football charity, and if I could support him getting the camp back up and running, then I'd feel a million bucks for it. I could see by his reaction that it meant a lot to him. The more I explained, the more he began realising that although it was a running adventure, there was a deeper meaning to it all. I wanted to do it for him too, and to contribute towards stroke awareness. It was a nice feeling knowing I was trying to do something he seemed proud of.

After my pitch, he knew I wasn't messing around, and it was something I was taking seriously. No matter how off the wall he thought the idea was, he was game to help me and needed no convincing. It was a weight off my shoulders.

Dad asked if I'd be willing to donate a portion to the National Rehabilitation Hospital, which had been instrumental in his recovery. How could I say no? If it made him happy, I was more than willing. The hospital team truly did provide exceptional care and support to him. Because of the NRH, he'd made an unexpectedly sharp bounce-back that Lazarus would tip his hat to. It was agreed, I decided to donate 80% to the Irish

Heart Foundation, 10% to the NRH and 10% to the Football Village of Hope.

After our chat, my dad insisted on driving me to the bus stop, at all hours of the morning, instead of letting me get a taxi.

'Don't be daft. It's not good for you to be doing that at silly o'clock. Get your sleep.'

'I'm not sleeping well these days anyway, and you're one to be talking about doing daft things,' Dad joked.

I knew once he said he would drive me, he would wake up and get into his car, no matter how much I tried to deter him.

Thick as thieves, we kept our scheming from the mammy a little while longer. No point upsetting her earlier than we had to. I waited four years until I broke the news to her about my first tattoo, so the timing had to be just right to trigger her catchphrase of mild motherly disapproval, 'Ah Alan'.

Like the online research and emails to Dean and Gerry, my chat with Dad could be seen as insignificant. But, like push starting a car, the first few steps can be the most challenging but the most important. Once I got moving, the steps became a bit easier. Before I knew it, I was off down the road, up and running. Verbalising my dream to my dad was me saying, *yes, this is happening*. It's no longer an internal whim, locked away in my head. I'm taking the necessary steps towards turning my vision into a reality by creating some expectation.

After my expedition to the midlands, I finally got to meet Gerry. It felt like a mini achievement, and I was quite chuffed with myself. I went from having the idea, doing my homework, contacting the expert in plenty of time, confiding in my dad, getting to the coffee shop meeting on time and now sitting down face to face with the man with the plan. It was all rewarding progress. Delighted with my map – and the reaction it got from Dad – I folded the enormous yoke out again. I showed Gerry the route I had planned, to prove that I had put some thought into this and was not just a timewaster. At the age of 20, most people don't have much life experience. All you can do is show enthusiasm, a willingness to learn, and a bit of initiative. You can only hope people more skilled and knowledgeable than you feel like mentoring you is a good investment of their time. I think he saw that in me, so he didn't disappoint and was willing to guide my enthusiasm.

Gerry explained how he and Ken raised €500,000. What made the event work from a fundraising perspective was that they organised 32 'mini-events' under the overarching challenge. Without a team of professional event organisers, they gave themselves a mountain of additional work, putting on 32 half and full-marathon races in each county and getting other runners involved. It required meticulous preparation: there were health and safety statements, first aid cover, public liability insurance, Garda clearances, road closures, water stations, race marshals, etc., to organise. Although hugely taxing, this additional undertaking enabled them to spread the fundraising responsibilities. Raising money for charity was an obligation now delegated to each runner, in each of the 32 race events. To take part, each runner would have to raise a minimum sum, contributing towards the overall event tally. It was much like you see in the London Marathon. Although you can enter London by paying €55 or so, the chances of getting a place are slim. Instead, thousands of people opt for a charity spot. Not only do you then have to pay the entry fee, but you also need to raise a minimum amount of money for the charity that chose you to represent them. This minimum can be upwards of €2,000. Thirty-two marathon events, with 32 participants, each raising an achievable €500, isn't long adding up to a phenomenal €500,000. It was a proven winning formula.

The thought of putting on participatory events around the coastline had never even crossed my mind. I had already bitten off more than I could chew. Since my ambition only stretched to running 42.2 kilometres solo, putting down a marker and returning the next day to repeat, there were fewer variables to worry about. I also didn't have to get there early and stay late to meet participants or have the time and effort of driving to a new county each day. I'd simply run and try to lay my head near to the finish/start line each day, keeping work time to a minimum and recovery to the maximum.

Gerry told me, 'Your approach will cut out so much added hassle and moving pieces. It will be much simpler from a logistics standpoint, and you can enjoy the running more.' Knowing my limited timeline and the work required for the running events that he had created, the fact that I was *only* running seemed to reassure him that I hadn't lost the plot – at least not entirely! Gerry talked me through his 22-week training plan, drawn up by Richard Donovan, a well-seasoned Irish international ultra-endurance runner. According to my Dean Karnazes book, the 'beginner's marathon training plan' was 26 weeks and the 'personal best marathon training plan' was 18 weeks. Most typical marathon training plans are 16 to 20 weeks long, so I was surprised and relieved that training for 35 consecutive marathons was in the same ballpark.

What the plan lacked in duration, it made up for in sheer volume. Most beginners aim to run at least one or two 'long runs' – typically around 32 kilometres – before showing up to a marathon run. My plan had about 20 long runs, many at the marathon 42.2 kilometres distance and a handful beyond it, up to 50 kilometres. The programme was, without a doubt, not for beginners. After all, my challenge would mean trying to run about 300 kilometres per week for five straight weeks. The training started with a hefty 80 kilometres to be covered in week one and progressively increased in weekly mileage to week 15. Week 15 was the peak of the training mountain, the plan expecting me to run a staggering 187 kilometres over seven days. It then 'tapered' down for seven weeks until it reached 64 kilometres in the least demanding week, just before the start of my challenge. When I say 'taper', 50% of those last few weeks of training still expected me to run over 145 kilometres per week. The taper period was to allow my damaged body to rebuild itself stronger, after getting torn to shreds climbing to the training peak. It didn't sound like easing off to me, but nonetheless, the purpose of the descent was to arrive at the start line healthy and in one piece, or so I was told by Gerry. I was happy to take his word for it and nodded in blind agreement. He emphasised that speed was not my friend and all these sessions were about accumulating long slow hours on my feet.

'That's great! Thanks very much for sharing it with me.'

I smiled in pure naivety, just delighted with myself for getting the action plan. I was ready to leave and hit the road. Gerry's eyebrows scrunched inward, and his mouth moved to one side, a perplexed look stared back at me. I think he was mistaking my blind youthful optimism about completing the training plan, for arrogance.

'By your unphased reaction, I take it you've done a lot of running so?'

'I have, yeah – years of it.' Like an unwanted question at a job interview, I was trying to say just enough to get by and hoping he wouldn't delve any deeper.

'What sort of mileage?'

Ah shite, I thought. 'Eh, I'm a sprinter by trade, so mileage hasn't been a staple. I'd do a five-kilometre run each week during the winter season, and we had to do cross country races growing up, but nothing like this madness. Oh, I did a 16-kilometre road run, but that was about six years ago now.'

'Riiiiight. Okay.' There was a pause. 'You're road running at the moment though, right?'

'Well, not really, no. I packed in sprinting last year and have just been hitting the weights.' Although the honest answer, I avoided eye contact, knowing it wasn't the correct answer.

Gerry started to look a bit concerned. 'You'd want to get going straight away on building up your distances before starting into this. You have about nine months, and this plan is just under six. It's not impossible, but you really should start now'. It was wise advice from an experienced ultra-distance athlete. *However*, I was booked to head off to Santa Ponsa in two weeks with two of my best friends. If I was going to be devoted to running solitary kilometres for months on end, I wanted to make the most of the little time left to enjoy my rare lack of training commitments. I respected Gerry and was grateful for his time, so the least I could do was be honest.

'I'm going to Spain in a few weeks with my friends. To me, there's not much point starting just to be stopping and starting again. After the holiday, I'll be locked into training camp until the run starts. I can assure you that.' I was accustomed to this process, but I think it made Gerry question my seriousness and ability to stay disciplined. He didn't seem too convinced or impressed with my approach but warmed to my hopeless optimism, nonetheless. He was an absolute gent. I owe him big time for sharing his valuable time with me.

Mission accomplished, I thought. I'd spoken to my dad and Gerry and did what I had to, to get the key. I had just about convinced Gerry to send me a copy of the blueprint he had followed. I was delighted, having solved a fundamental piece of the puzzle. The small success was more fuel to keep moving.

SINK TO SWIM

When I got my teeth into Gerry's book, I discovered the final test of endurance he set himself before committing to his 32-marathon challenge: completing a double Ironman. The race consisted of two 3.9-kilometre swims, two 180-kilometre cycles and two 42.2-kilometre runs. I had already committed to my challenge, with no endurance experience, but thought it would be no harm to try to replicate the man's method. I wasn't a total idiot, so I didn't go sign up for an Ironman with no training – never mind a double Ironman. While ordering fish and chips, I spotted a poster for a humble sprint triathlon planned for Tramore. It was a week away, so I thought, *that'll do grand*. This was meagre compared to Gerry's test. The sprint triathlon consisted of a 750-metre sea swim, a 20-kilometre cycle and a five-kilometre beach run. It's all relative, though. By that stage, Gerry was an experienced endurance athlete. I hadn't swum in donkeys' years and had a week to prepare – which mainly consisted of finding a loan of a bicycle and a wetsuit. I felt no desire to try to outdo Gerry. A sprint triathlon was probably about as testing for me then, as the gigantic triathlon was for his well-trained body. You can only start from where you are, and it shouldn't devalue the effort because someone else can do more or better.

I was pretty blasé about the triathlon. I oversimplified it, which I'd pick any day instead of overcomplicating and overthinking things. I'd much rather be let loose on a climbing wall to fall and climb again than spend hours learning the theory of climbing and where's best to put your foot in this and that hypothetical situation. Just let me at it. For me, oversimplifying means I try before I'm necessarily ready. 'Ready' rarely exists, so best to get on with trying and learning. The likely outcome is that I fall flat on my face, but quick failure feedback provides an opportunity for fast learning. Overcomplicating things leads to paralysis by analysis. As Bruce Lee said, 'If you want to learn to swim, jump into the water. On dry land, no frame of mind is ever going to help you.'

I thought, *How hard can a little triathlon really be? You*

were a sprinter for years. Five kilometres? That'll be grand! Isn't the saying, it's as easy as riding a bike and sure don't you cycle two kilometres to work and back? Sorted. You took swimming lessons for six years straight. Not a bother to you, Al! I failed to appreciate eight years had passed since I quit swimming, and the passing of time can make a bit of a difference.

That last one was indeed an error of judgement on my part, but live and learn, eh? With no time to prepare, I hit the pool on Monday, intending to cover the full 750-metre distance in one slow, relaxed go. This pool rehearsal was meant to put my mind at ease in advance of having to do it in the sea, surrounded by other participants. Gasping for air after just two lousy lengths of the pool, I had to stop. This was no 50-metre Olympic pool either; it was only a 20-metre hotel pool. I was screwed! Once I could breathe again, I started the breaststroke. Given my unrealistic expectations, this was embarrassing. Breaststroke was for the older, unfit people in the slow lane. After one rosy-cheeked length, I reverted to something resembling the front crawl for the next length. My inefficiency zapped all my oxygen. *This method will have to do.* I swam breaststroke and 'front crawl' on rotation and stopped for air when I had to but eventually got the distance done. I was so exhausted from the flailing, I needed the next day off. On Wednesday, I repeated my attempt with the same concerning result. I never recalled swimming being anywhere near as hard. I was like a stone. I took Thursday and Friday to rest, or 'taper off', as Gerry had taught me, before the race on Saturday. I couldn't string 40 metres of front crawl together in the pool before needing to stop. I had failed miserably on my two attempts to cover the sprint triathlon distance in practice.

My friend Seán Drohan reassured me. He was lending me his surf wetsuit for the event. He advised me it would act as a buoyancy aid and make the swim much more manageable than my experiences wearing baggy shorts in the pool. Armed with that glimmer of hope, I was stubbornly going to give it a lash.

I may have won All-Ireland medals, but I felt awfully out of place rocking up to the triathlon. It was an educational experience, going from being a seasoned juvenile competitor to being an absolute beginner and a hazard to the mostly middle-aged racers – a fish out of water. I was literally the only person with chunky bicycle wheels, having borrowed my brother's bike and got it serviced that week. Everyone else had slick racing bikes with stick-thin tires. My outlier status was reinforced by being the only person in a surf wetsuit; everyone else had much more expensive swim specific wetsuits. I looked like a right plonker, but what can you do! I was there, so no turning back.

Something I hadn't thought about until I was at the start line, staring out to sea, was how I was going to navigate the crowd once we all hit the water at the same time. Admittedly, landing yourself in a spot of bother is a slight pitfall of the jump first ask questions later attitude. At this late stage, I could only smile at the situation I had put myself in. *This should be interesting.*

The buzzer sounded, and we were sprinting enthusiastically towards the waves. The swarm of swimmers quickly answered my question. Everyone who could swim just bulldozed through me as I got struck by arms and legs from all angles. I was gasping for air at the best of times in the serene leisure centre. Now in the sea, where the air should have been was salty water, as competitors kicked, stroked and splashed aggressively. Not only was I being deprived of oxygen, my vision was a mix of fogged up goggles, swinging baseball bats of neoprene and buckets of water being chucked at my face. My line of travel was impossible to gauge amongst the pandemonium. It was feckin' lethal stuff altogether!

When the competitive swimmers had zoomed ahead of me and having lived to tell the tale of the initial shemozzle, I sighed relief. I had some space to gasp for air towards the back of the pack, reverting to doing the breaststroke, which demanded less oxygen. To say I nearly drowned isn't much of an overstatement. I was backstroking, breaststroking and doing something slightly similar to a front crawl, but I was moving forwards, nonetheless. I couldn't hold my breath long enough to put my head in the sea. My peculiar racing style warranted concern from the event's safety kayakers.

'Are you okay? Do you want to hold onto the kayak for a minute?'

'I'm. Grand. Don't. Worry. About. Me.' I huffed in staccato.

What a joy to get onto the beach. The *firma* the surface, the less the *terra*! I wanted to sit down and celebrate being alive, but crowds were watching, and Dad was there cheering me on, so I had to huff and puff my way to the bicycle area. Only a few bikes were left, so there was zero hassle finding my clunky yoke. It was nice to be able to sit down, the secure pavement beneath my wheels a welcome change from the inhospitable sea. I was left so far behind in the swim that I was able to gain places in the cycle, despite the state of the bike, zero training and dropping my drink in the first few hundred yards, fumbling for the holder like a newbie.

Enthusiastically stepping off the bike, my legs were like jelly once planted on the ground. It was so strange moving from one discipline to the other for the first time, calling on different muscles. It took a few hundred metres for my body to realise what was going on, and then I settled into a nice running pace, picking people off, sprinting in to secure a mid-table finish.

My triathlon experience was no confidence boost, like the one Gerry got and needed before committing to his consecutive marathon challenge. It was a good thing that I didn't use this as a test to decide if I had what it took to run 35 marathons back-to-back. I had told Dad I would do it, and I had motivation. That was enough for me. A silver lining in the ordeal was that it proved I was willing to flounder in water, rather than admit defeat. It wasn't pretty, but I got it done. That's the attitude this marathon run would need. Times wouldn't be an indicator of success or failure, just the ability to show up and finish the distance mattered. Attitude would be everything.

NO REST FOR THE WICKED

With Gerry Duffy's training plan in hand and my dismal performance in the shortened triathlon, I knew I'd be screwed if I jumped straight into his training programme, starting with 80 kilometres in week one. With the challenge due to commence towards the end of May, Gerry's training regimen wouldn't begin until the end of December, so I had some time to train for the training. I needed help to bridge the gap and get my novice ass in shape in the limited time I had available. At the same time as reaching out to Gerry Duffy, I had contacted a long-distance coach in my old athletics club, Gerry Deegan. He had competed for Ireland at the World Cross Country Championships numerous times and was lightning quick – recording a marathon time of 2 hours and 18 minutes in the eighties. Luckily this Gerry was local. He was kind enough to give up his time to me and was intrigued by my initial pitch.

As we sat on my living room couch and he listened to my plans, he thought it was crackers – especially as he knew me as a sprinter. Over everything else, he was apprehensive about the conditions I'd set for myself. No rest days was bonkers, in his expert opinion. It was entirely up to me he said, but he strongly encouraged me to reconsider this aspect. In my head, it just sounded better as a donation plea. That was reason enough to roll with it. Doing 35 marathons in 35 days, to raise €35,000, seemed much catchier than 35 marathons in 40 days. I thought the days off would prolong the suffering, slow momentum and add a week of extra crew, physio, food, and accommodation costs to the logistics puzzle too. That would mean more variables, which were more things that might scupper the attempt. I think Gerry thought it more than a bit foolhardy and it's certainly hard to disagree with his logic. I just reassured Gerry that I wasn't deluded enough to be thinking of going anywhere near what he would consider marathon pace.

'Think of it more as 35 very long recovery runs, Gerry. There's no better time to say it's a marathon, not a sprint.' I assured him I would be extremely cautious with the speed of each and every marathon.

'Right. Well, I still think you're mad but glad to be of assistance.'

He still wasn't convinced after my attempts at reassurance, knowing more than most about the toll a marathon has on the body. Despite his concern for my wellbeing, he wanted to give me the best opportunity at succeeding. He devised a short training programme so I could build up to the start line of Gerry Duffy's intimidating plan. The blueprint was now all there in black and white and colour coded squares. It was up to me to execute the plan to the best of my ability.

HALF-BAKED IDEA

After returning from a week of excessive drinking in Spain, towards the end of September 2011, I was in no fit shape to be running but had no time to feel sorry for myself with my hangover. I had to dust off the trainers, pull up the socks and get moving.

The sprint triathlon wasn't my only bright idea. Sure, it gave me a picture of the poor shape I was in, but it wasn't a real litmus test. Before starting the training plans, I signed myself up for the Dublin Marathon. As with the short triathlon, I gave myself little to no time to prepare. The race was four weeks out, at the end of October. Using the word loosely, I thought it would be 'wise' to experience at least one marathon, before starting training and declaring I'd be running 35 of them in 35 days come May. I needed to discover what I was getting myself into first.

Most people would think preparing for and running one marathon, or running 101 marathons, would be the course of action to take *before* signing up to my challenge. It's hard to argue. I think that the sensible approach would have equipped me with too much knowledge and ammunition to back away from my challenge. It would also take years to amass the level of experience required to be considered qualified to try. I was where I was and had no notions of changing course now. I would just need to continue on the path I'd locked myself into.

Running a marathon would be the best way to discover where the baseline was and focus my mind on the challenges ahead. I hadn't learned from my triathlon near-drowning experience and was lackadaisical in my preparation for the Dublin Marathon too. I just thought I could rock up and complete it with relative ease. I thought back on the 16 kilometres I ran with no distance training. It was easy fun. *The marathon shouldn't be much different, right?* Wrong again.

I naively set out on my self-created four-week couch to marathon programme. I had to create one because, despite all the information available online, apparently, a four-week marathon training plan is not a thing. My invention consisted of three weeks to build up to one long and slow 29-kilometre run. Having learned from the pro, I allowed myself one easy week, in the end, to taper. *Very sensible and measured.* I was truly flying by the seat of my pants, but I was fine with it. If anything, I was feeling pretty confident going into the marathon; I had achieved a new personal best, running 29-kilometres in the lead-up – the furthest I'd ever moved on foot. There was no injury or pain, and I didn't keel over. I didn't know what the fuss was about. *Stepping from 29-kilometres to 42.2-kilometres will be grand,* I thought.

CHARITY

During the ill-conceived preparation period for my first ever marathon, I met with the Irish Heart Foundation. It was the 28th September 2011, the start of my fourth and final college year. The initial meeting was a great success, as I made my commitment to run a lap of Ireland in a few months. Their senior fundraising professional loved the idea. He saw a lot of potential in it, especially when I told them about Gerry and Ken's triumph, with the hundreds of thousands they raised with a shorter challenge.

Being aware that my dad was a former President of the Football Association of Ireland, he jumped at the opportunity to capitalise.

'Might you discuss with your dad, the possibility of gaining access to the Aviva Stadium for the charity's volunteers to do a bucket collection, in the build-up to your run and to Euro 2012?' I thought it was a fantastic idea. *Why didn't I think of that?* I guess that's why they're paid the big bucks! 'If you can get us the permission to go inside the stadium on a match day, the Heart Foundation will sort the rest: volunteers and Garda permits to collect on the streets around it too. A stadium and street collection on match day would be amazing.'

Great, I thought. *The charity is fully behind my initiative, adding helpful ideas of their own and promising bodies to make the most of the fundraising opportunity.* The stadium collection could be thousands of euro raised before even running a step around Ireland, purely on the promise of the run at a future date. The more the fundraising professional spoke, the more I was at ease with the likelihood of raising tens of thousands of euros.

I handed them my overly ambitious training plan, made them aware that I was in the final year of my degree, and worked part-time in Waterford on weekends.

'This is going to be a full-on few months for me.'

Truth be told, between Dad's stroke in March and this September meeting, I hadn't put much if any thought into the logistics and the cost aspect of the project. I was too preoccupied trying to resolve the training conundrum. Having the Heart Foundation meeting forced me to take a more holistic event-organiser approach, rather than a singular runner's approach. I was a college boy, and he was a suited and booted paid professional. I needed to demonstrate to them that I had at least considered what I was getting myself in for beyond *just* running.

Once again, I folded out and showed off my beloved map and explained the rules I'd set for myself. 'Each day I'll run 42.2 kilometres, stick down a marker and return to the same point the next day, to run a further 42.2 kilometres, until I circumnavigate the island. I'll be running from Waterford, where I'm from, back to Waterford, the scenic route. Simple as that.'

I'd need to get a website up so the public can find out about the challenge, the three charities and how to make donations. I'd need a support vehicle and volunteers to help me around the route. I'd need to try to arrange accommodation and three meals a day for the team and me. Ideally, I'd have a physio session after each marathon, and I'd need to try to find a gear sponsor, particularly for runners. I found advice telling me to change them every 500 kilometres or so, to reduce the risk of injury. I had over 4,000 kilometres to complete during training and the event itself.

That meant at least eight pairs of runners.

With trainers costing around €150 a pop, it's not long adding up. Throw in 35 nights of accommodation and 35 days of food for the two-person crew and me, plus 35 physio sessions and a support vehicle, and you're easily over €15,000 in costs. I was a minimum wage kitchen porter, working 15 hours a week. I certainly couldn't afford it. Gerry Duffy, Ken Whitelaw and Eddie Izzard all raised hundreds of thousands, and Terry Fox raised millions. *Surely, it'll be handy enough to get some corporate backing in exchange for positive publicity for being associated with this Irish based charity endurance adventure.*

The Heart Foundation representative was of the same thinking as me. To my delight, he assured me the charity would organise the logistics. 'You worry about getting your degree and all the training done, and we'll sort the rest. Just confirm where you'll be finishing each day. It's the least we can do for all your efforts.'

That was huge for me. The offer of that level of support was unexpected, much appreciated and needed. It seemed a fair arrangement given the thousands of kilometres and hours I would need to put in to prepare, running for their financial gain, on top of my work and final year study commitments. We shook hands in agreement, both 'delira and excira' with our day's work. I left the charity's office skipping out the door, confident I could hold up my end of the bargain and optimistic about the professional's excitement and commitment. My mind was at ease.

DUBLIN MARATHON

Now that I had all the chips pushed firmly to the centre of the table, the time had come to actually run a marathon and see what the craic was all about.

I was renting with two other students in Stoneybatter, in Dublin City Centre at the time. On the 31st October 2011, I hopped on the Luas to join the crowds on Fitzwilliam Street Upper, at the Dublin Marathon's start line. I was apprehensive, like before a test I hadn't studied for, but the crowds and buzz of anticipation nullified the nerves with adrenaline. The skies were clear on this fresh morning, my breath visible in the air. In the shade of the Georgian red-brick terraces, I was kept lukewarm by a tatty jumper and tracksuit bottoms over my running shorts and t-shirt.

The start gun blasted, and I hurriedly discarded my decrepit outer shell on a railing. I had no idea of pacing, so I just headed off at what felt sensible. I should have known better from my sprint days; what feels like a leisurely pace on the first sprint, can feel impossible by sprint number 10.

By the halfway mark, I wasn't in a good place at all, at all, and had significant doubts, with 21 kilometres still left to run. *This is not nice.* With 15 kilometres left, I was becoming feral, mentally stripped back, the pains were growing, and I was getting emotional from the encouragement of the strangers lining the roadside. I specifically remember a guy in a wheelchair, holding a sign saying something along the lines of 'keep running for me'. Jesus, he had me fighting back the tears. I was in a downward spiral. Trying to spit (disgusting, I know), it landed on my t-shirt, but I couldn't have given less of a feck how I looked at this stage. Without the pleasure of being drunk, I imagined I looked like a fella after 10 pints, jacket hanging off, lost wallet, fixated on trudging off-balance like a zombie to bed, with taxi after taxi passing him. This was proper fight or flight stuff, as the toll of the effort was accumulating. I felt I had as good a chance of running to the horizon as I did of getting to the damn finish line.

I was in a much better headspace once the 42.2-kilometre finish line seemed in reach. *That's 35 kilometres, 36 kilometres ... we're getting there, Al, yes boy.* It proves the power and importance of my thoughts. My muscles, tendons and joints were fine at the start, screaming in the middle and then feeling better near the end. Logically, they had to be getting more beat up as the kilometres clocked up. The only reason it felt easier was that I knew I was going to finish. I had come through 37 kilometres, so what's another five? Even at the worst of times when there was no light at the end of the tunnel, I knew it would appear at some point if I kept moving. *You've gone through too much just to give in now; you got this!* I told myself.

I felt part of something bigger than just me. The supporters were cheering and holding out Jelly Babies and tubs of Vaseline. Runners too were patting other runners on the back if their demeanour was looking negative. Re-entering the city centre, I was fully bought into the powerful experience and on a high. I was converted.

'You're doing great, nearly there, bud,' I said, encouraging some random lad who had slowed, looking like me a few kilometres earlier. We were in this struggle together, and we were going to make it through together.

'Fuckin' hell,' was the exclamation of relief when I crossed the line in Merrion Square in a time of 4 hours and 13 minutes. The lowest I'd ever placed in anything I'd entered – 5,723rd place, out of 11,245 runners but slightly faster than the day's average time of 4 hours and 19 minutes. I was in too much of a state to care. I was done and needed to get my ass to bed as soon as possible before I collapsed.

I had only told my immediate family and my flatmate Simon Cody about the run. I hadn't made any fuss of it at all. I told them, 'It's not a big deal; I'm just off for a jog.' I wished I had hammed it up when I saw family and friends swarming their loved ones at the finish. Not for any egotistical reasons, but for the sheer practicality of having someone to meet at the finish line with warm and dry clothes; someone to help hold my body upright and escort me home in one piece. It was a bit of an oversight. Naively, I thought there wouldn't be a bother on me, expecting to skip home. I hadn't anticipated being a broken shadow of myself.

I wrapped myself up like a turkey at Christmas in the complimentary finisher's foil blanket, in an attempt to retain some heat. The crowds of runners and onlookers, coupled with my banjaxed body, restricted me to a snail's pace, as I tried to hobble my way to the Luas stop. All I desperately wanted was to be warm, dry and horizontal. I looked pitiful. I knew because of the way by-passers were looking at me, pulling their lips inwards, raising their eyebrows and giving me a short nod, as if to say, *There, there, you'll be alright, young fella.* I certainly did not feel okay as my rain, and sweat-soaked shorts and t-shirt stuck uncomfortably to my now shivering fragile body, as I gingerly shuffled forward. *Ow! Why can't these fuckers move so I can get home?*

I eventually inched to the Luas stop, off O'Connell Street. My suspicion was correct. Catching my reflection in the tram's window, I looked nothing like what I suspected a successful marathon finisher should look like. I looked like a miserable drowned rat, with a wet head of hair, hugging myself with the tinfoil sheet.

When I eventually reached the flat, I whacked the shower to boiling and must have sat in the corner for 30 minutes, eyes closed and head resting against the wall – a sorry sight. I had intended to have one last bank holiday blowout before taking a day off and starting my training plan. Somewhat brought back to the land of the living after the long warm shower, I cracked open a bottle of cider with Simon. I got halfway through it and had to go for a strategic nap, so I'd be able for a few celebratory evening scoops. That plan went out the window, as I woke up over 10 hours later, in even more agony than before, delayed-onset muscle soreness (DOMS) in full effect. It was more like delayed-onset bone soreness. I was very used to muscle soreness, mainly tight calves, hamstrings or glutes, from my days of football and sprinting, but I'd never experienced my shins, knees, heels and hips being in smithereens before. I felt like I had been dump tackled by Paul O'Connell, with his full weight crushing my lower body. I was so sore I only left the bed the next day to shuffle to the bathroom, which felt like too much movement to be attempting. Simon threw me in a bit of grub to sustain me, as I lay in a woeful heap in bed all day, thinking about what was to come in the months ahead.

The brutal reality of marathon running had well and truly set in, along with a fair degree of concern. Better late than never, I suppose. At least I knew what my baseline was now and what to expect if I ran with no foundation at all. The house would unceremoniously crumble in an instant. That knowledge would stand me in good stead and scare me into building a mighty foundation capable of withstanding any endurance challenge.

I was due to meet with the charity fundraiser at the Irish Heart Foundation office again, the Thursday after the marathon. He was going to introduce me to his colleague, the Communications Manager, who was going to help with the fundraising drive.

After the run, on Sunday, I was dead to the world on Monday, and still bedridden with aches and pains on Tuesday. This type of suffering is reserved for fools, like me, who tried to ignore the laws of science and paid the full price. By Wednesday, I tried to walk the 10 minutes to college, got halfway there and decided to retreat, doing the limp of shame back to bed. I thought, *What are they going to think of me if I show up to the charity office in this sorry state, after just one marathon.*

Although broken, I couldn't cancel the Thursday meeting. What impression would that give? The best solution was to whack a load of Paracetamol into me and to try to put on an unphased mask.

'Good morning. What's the strongest pain killer you have, please?'

The pharmacist was duly suspicious with my needy

opening line. I had to explain the marathon and severe joint pains. Thankfully she obliged, and I was on the bus to the southside of Dublin. When I made it to the charity's office in Ballsbridge, I stopped at the door and took a deep breath. *Walk normally, suck up the pain and don't look like an idiot,* I told myself. I didn't want to give them cause for concern or reason to withdraw their offer of help, or worse yet, back out entirely, not wanting to be associated with a doomed project.

'We're going to go to the coffee shop down the road today, if that's alright, Alan?'

You dicks, I thought, of the wholly innocent, pleasant and polite employees. My body still hurt so bad.

'Yeah, sounds great. You lead the way ... Is it far?'

I just about held myself together for the excruciating walk. It was another uplifting meeting with the two keen charity professionals. I left with further reassurances that I should focus on getting permission for the stadium bucket collection, completing my marathon training, and passing my final year at college. I'd also need to find a two-person support team to accompany me for the duration of the five-week tour. Other than that, the charity had my back and would sort the rest – corporate sponsors, sponsored running gear, sponsored accommodation and food, sponsored physios, a support vehicle on loan, an event website page and generating positive media coverage to fuel donations to the charity.

CRIPPLED

Given my body's state after running just one marathon,

particularly my knees, I was understandably questioning how I was going to get my body to hold up for 35 consecutive marathons. I wasn't having doubts about going through with it at all. In my mind, I was fully resigned to running, walking or crawling, if needs be, to get each 42.2-kilometre section done. I had 24 hours to cover the marathon distance. I knew I'd only fail if I was incapacitated or could not physically cover the distance in a day, despite giving every ounce of strength. Although I was willing to go there, I didn't want it to be so torturous. It was no joke struggling to walk for three-plus days after the Dublin Marathon. *How am I going to run another marathon and another marathon, for five weeks straight?* I was naive enough to start this thing and just needed to be stubborn enough to prepare for war and see it out to the finish. Running an entire lap of Ireland seemed like a pipedream at this moment, but focusing on how hard it would be, wasn't going to get the challenge done. As my friend Ben Clerkin would say, 'You're making obstacles out of opportunities!' With an evidently awful baseline of marathon fitness, there was a huge opportunity to make quick and significant gains in my endurance capabilities.

With the training plan just kicking off and the debilitating pain of my one measly marathon fresh in my mind, and still lingering throughout my body, I booked in for an appointment with a physiotherapist. I was in for a sports massage and gait analysis. The analysis involved walking over a mat with sensors noting abnormalities in how I planted my foot. The gizmo detected where I was distributing my weight, and two custom shoe insoles, called orthotics, were produced to correct the imbalances.

Orthotics are a heavily debated topic. One argument is that

they align your feet to land correctly and help reduce suffering and injury risk. The other view is that they are like putting your foot in a cast, artificially providing a quick fix, rather than correcting the root of the problem. If your arm wasn't functioning right, would you just wrap some plaster of Paris around it every time you needed to use it, or would you do mobility, flexibility and strength work to make it self-sufficient? Probably the latter. However, time was not in abundance, and I was desperate for a quick fix to relieve the knee pain. I went for the orthotic band-aid, rather than spending a year plus trying to correct my weaknesses.

NUTRITION

At the same time, I sought out nutritional advice. I paid Barry Murray to steer me. He has a Masters in Sports and Exercise Nutrition from Loughborough University and was a competitive international ultra-distance runner himself. I had to complete a food diary, noting all the drinks and food I consumed over a week-long period so that he could dissect my habits.

I've always been tall and bony, finding it hard to gain mass. I was lean at the time, less than 11% body fat but slightly bulkier than in my scrawny endurance sprinting days. With no track sessions or competition season to worry about, I enjoyed packing on some meat in the weights room, so my frame had filled out a little in the year since quitting athletics.

I was surprised when he said I should lose some weight. Although I enjoyed the extra time in the gym and it helped my confidence, it was counterproductive to my new goal. I was lean, but I guess not optimal distance runner lean. Over longer distances, it pays to be lighter on the feet and kinder to the impacted joints. Take one look at the elites who line up at the start of any marathon, and you'll know what I mean about an efficient endurance athlete's build.

No crazy diet for me, though. The weight would fall off following my demanding training schedule. If anything, I'd be eating more to fuel the training and struggling not to waste away. I just kept it simple as I always had and stuck to whole, unprocessed foods as much as possible. It didn't need to be rocket science. If I ate lots of fast food and sugary junk food, my health would suffer. I never completely eliminated junk food, or even alcohol, but kept them to a sparse minimum, maybe 5-10% of my calorie intake – not that I ever monitored it. In training, this meant the odd three pints with friends, fish and chips here and there or a treat of Minstrels and Coke for a movie night. With the demands I would be putting on myself, I needed to treat my body the best I could and give it the finest fuel, but there was certainly no need for any of this 'cheat meal' craic or unsustainable restrictions. I just enjoyed what I wanted to eat or drink and was responsible and accountable enough for my own wellbeing, not acting the maggot at either extreme.

There were no major shakeups. My main tips from the expert were drinking more water and preparing snacks between main meals, like peanut butter and oatcakes, or fruit and nuts. He suggested eating more on big mileage days and less on low mileage days and having my main meal directly after my workout to enhance my recovery. I learned a nifty trick to replicate energy gels I couldn't afford too: take an empty vitamin tablet tube, lob in a bit of honey, salt and a shot of hot water; Bob's your uncle; a pinch of coffee too, for a caffeinated energy gel. On my restricted student budget, I was all for penny-pinching solutions. The meeting was worth it for the oatcakes and peanut butter tip alone – a filling, budget-friendly staple snack ever since.

RUNNING WILD

Living in Stoneybatter, I was blessed with my proximity to the Phoenix Park – an ideal playground for an aspiring ultra-distance runner. While saving up for a GPS watch, I had to make do with counting roundabouts at the start. It made training a bit dreary: two kilometres from my flat to roundabout one, three-point-five kilometres to roundabout two, five kilometres to roundabout three and five-point-five kilometres to the end of the park. It did the job, but I struggled with the monotony of the route. When it didn't conveniently line up with those exact distances, I'd have to pre-plan the run and jog between certain roundabouts a certain number of times.

I eventually scrubbed enough pots and pans to be able to splurge on a GPS watch for my birthday in December. It gave me the freedom to head off-piste onto the dirt trails, making things so much easier. Not physically – the ground was uneven with mud, puddles and sprawling tree roots, but it just felt good to be amidst nature. I escaped order, the mind-numbing and soul-destroying concrete path which shot straight as an arrow from one end of the park to the other, under artificial street lights and subject to the noise and fumes of vehicle traffic. The trails were wild, and each run felt like an exciting micro-adventure.

I'll never forget my first encounter with the park's resident stags. It was around 07:00 a.m. and I was five kilometres in, when standing directly in front of me was a large stag. He stared straight at me, not giving an inch, pointing his intimidating antlers towards the sky for me to appreciate their full glory. I froze on the path like a rabbit in the headlights. This scenario had never crossed my mind until that moment, and I had no idea about these wild animals' temperament. *Is he going to ram me? I should have looked into this. Ehhh ...*

'Good stag, that's a good boy,' I said calmly, as I slowly gave him a wide berth, showing him my palms in peace, moving off the worn trail and into the soggy overgrown grass, primed to sprint if needed.

Once I was a safe distance past him, I was beaming for the rest of the run. The day hadn't even started for most students, and there I was, having this wilderness experience in my backyard. I felt like I had the park to myself, taking in the twittering dawn chorus, scampering under the mature tree cover. I could have been in any remote destination in the world, not in the centre of a capital city.

COMMUNITY SUPPORT

Although the Irish Heart Foundation advised me to focus solely on the demanding physical preparation and complete my final year at college, I was working on more ways to generate money for them and the other two charities. One idea was to ask my childhood football club, Tramore AFC, if they could do something to assist, like run a small tournament.

I knew I had to start telling people what I was up to sooner or later; this meant things were getting more serious. First on my hit list were Tramore AFC's head honchos, Paul Power, my first football coach, and John Power, the club's chairman. I played with the club for a decade, and Dad had been a regular in the clubhouse for tea, biscuits and a chat about all things football. It was as good a place as any to start putting myself and my dream out there. With my dad beside me, I gave the men the run down.

'Are you mad?' they both said simultaneously, with a grin.

Dad was cracking up, hearing the plan aloud again and seeing the lad's reaction. It was fun seeing the response – the surprise, concern, intrigue and enthusiasm all at once and in equal parts.

I had to brazenly tell people my ambition and risk the reputational damage if I failed to at least cover a respectable distance in the summer. I say brazen since I only had one average marathon under my belt and I had been hobbling for days after the shaggin' thing. I hadn't yet earned the right to make such brash statements. Sharing ambitions aloud to people shouldn't be underestimated in its difficulty and its potentially powerful effect. The more people I told, the more pressure there was and the more responsibility I felt to deliver on my word.

'I'm running a lap of Ireland.'

The more people I confided my dream in, the more it became a reality. I was adding fuel to my fire and fanning it.

Paul, who had diligently devoted his life to coaching football in Tramore, voiced his concern about the toll the run would have on my body. He knew I wasn't messing around with my intent and preparation though, and I managed to reassure him. They assured me they'd be delighted if the club could help and said to leave it with them.

Not only did the inaugural Tramore AFC Christmas fundraising football blitz raise about €2,000 towards my run's fundraising total, but it's also done this for other causes, year in and year out ever since. Although the dedicated club members did all the hard work, I feel proud to have been the spark to initiate and help establish this growing community tradition. Participant numbers and the money raised have steadily increased, all to the credit of the club and the local community. This show of support from my club gave me a morale boost to continue ploughing on with my solitary runs. Without even reaching the start line, I had funds to donate from my ambitious words and initiative alone. *I better not let them all down now,* I thought.

With the football fundraiser coming up, I had to tell my mother before she heard it from someone else. As expected, Mam wanted me to err on the side of caution with a seemingly safer pastime.

'What about your knees? All that running on the road: you'll hurt yourself. Would you not stick with the sprinting?'

'That ship's sailed, Mam. I wasn't enjoying it anymore and sprinting wouldn't raise a tap. Anyway, how many people get injured each year doing that? Loads!'

'Well, what about doing a triathlon then or the London Marathon? Wouldn't that be challenging enough, and you wouldn't be pounding your joints on the roads as much?'

'Triathlon doesn't interest me. I want to run around

Ireland and raise a bomb for charity while doing it. A man has got to do, what a man has got to do,' I quoted from the 1993 film *Cool Runnings*, when Junior followed his Olympic Jamaican bobsleigh dreams against his father's wishes.

Mam was worried and wanted to protect me. I got it. She wasn't wrong about the risk of damage, but the run wasn't up for debate. I was obsessed with the all-consuming pursuit by then. At 20, I didn't want to live a life in the security of the harbour. There would be no fun or satisfaction in playing it small and safe. I didn't see the point in being able-bodied but showing ingratitude for this gift by not pushing my limits. I felt the ultra-endurance run could make a more meaningful impact than sprinting or triathlon, and it excited me much more. I knew Mam would come around once she saw my passion and dedication, despite her fear and hesitation. It was a weight off my mind to tell her. She at least knew what Dad and I were up to now, so there was no more sneaking about.

JUGGLE

By December 2011, I was in full-on juggling mode. My Run Diary entry from the 8th December tells me that I was up and at it for an hour of strength work in the gym from 08:30 a.m., then straight to college to work on my final year project until 06:30 p.m. After a rushed dinner, I was off with friends to a Lisa Hannigan and James Vincent McMorrow gig in Temple Bar until about midnight. The fun wasn't over. There was still a two-hour journey home to Waterford and the day's run left to squeeze in. Sneaking in the door, I started lacing and layering up as quietly as I could.

Dad still wasn't sleeping much after the stroke and left the bed to see what the craic was. He was surprised to see me changing into my running gear. I looked at my watch – 02:00 a.m.

'You're cracked. Well, enjoy, I guess,' giving my dedication the nod of approval.

With eight kilometres pencilled in, I was off out Waterford's ring road, feeling like Rocky, with my full tracksuit and woolly hat on, hood up, watching my breath steam out in the dark, frosty air.

I passed a man walking his dog, and thought, *You lunatic, what are you doing out here walking at this hour of the morning? Go back to bed for yourself.* With some self-reflection, I had to laugh at myself for being in the same loony box as him.

Collapsing into bed at 03:00 a.m., I decided I needed to say 'no' more and prioritise training and recovery. I got the work done, but this burning of the candle at both ends had to stop.

UP AND AT 'EM

By Monday the 26th December, I had the Dublin Marathon in the bank and a few grand in donations for the three charities. I had also completed Gerry Deegan's starter training block, which laid a foundation of fitness. The knee pains had started to subside, with the measured, structured and consistent increase in weekly distance. The support of the orthotics was helping too, I felt. With Santa having delivered a CamelBak hydration backpack, it was time to start proper ultra-distance training and hop on the treadmill of Gerry Duffy's daunting 22-week programme. I knew things would not relent until it was time to put my toe on the start line in May, when things would get gravely serious: five consecutive 295-kilometre weeks of running.

I wasn't focusing on the incomprehensible distance of the challenge. I knew it would be won or lost in repeating the small mundane daily effort. My blinkers needn't splay wider than seven days, and the big picture will look after itself in due course. I could easily get overwhelmed with the magnitude of it all otherwise.

The initial months of work were such a period of growth. I had been consistently training five to seven times a week in my sprinting days, just to shave fractions of one second off my times, or even get slower some years. I forgot what it was like to start from scratch. As a beginner distance runner, the leaps and bounds made during the start of my transformation were exhilarating. I embraced being godawful at first. I knew I had to start from where I was – a useless distance runner – and knew where I was heading – Forrest Gump. With each passing day of small effort, I could feel my ability improving: a white belt slowly beating a challenger at a time, fighting towards a black belt.

The great thing I found about distance running was the accessibility of it. It started at my doorstep. While I was used to putting in three hours of commute and warm-up time for 15 minutes of beneficial quality sprint training, I just had to get out my door, and the valuable endurance work started accumulating. No time wasted.

Completing mundane daily tasks was much harder than it sounded though. I had many a battle with my inner weaknesses, especially during my initial winter weeks of training. The real challenge was not running 35 marathons in May and June when donations were rolling in, and people were encouraging me. The challenge lay in getting my inexperienced backside out of bed in December, January and February; running kilometres on my own in the frost, wind and rain. As Muhammad Ali said, 'The fight is won far from the witnesses, behind the lines, in the gym, and out there on the road; long before I dance under those lights.'

Unlike my football and sprinting days, no team or coach expected and depended on me to show up. I was accountable to nobody else. The alarm would be set, and I'd go to sleep with the best of intentions for the following morning. The buzzer would rudely wake me at the crack of dawn. In my pitch-black room, wrapped in my toasty duvet, with my head snuggled in the soft pillow, I'd hear the wind howling and that lovely Irish sideways rain pelting my window. I'd perform a split-second calculation in favour of being lazy. *Aw, you don't want to get out of bed to run for hours in that shitty weather alone. You have a rest day Thursday and a rest day Saturday. If you sleep in now, you can make it up then.* With haste and one eye open and the other squinting, I'd readjust my phone's alarm to give me just enough time to make my first lecture, and I'd go back snoring.

At the initial stage of training, I could get away with hitting the snooze button on a Monday with no problem. I was doing myself no favours, as the programme was designed as it was for a reason: so I'd run, recover, run, recover, etc. My method of recover, recover, recover, and then cram all my training towards the back end of the week was plain stupid. I'd run the full distance I was supposed to for the week, but by deferring it all to the end of the week, it was far from optimal for my progress and health.

Soon though, rest days disappeared from the schedule and every day would involve at least an eight-kilometre run to keep the engine improving. I knew I had to do something to break this bad habit of being a lazy git at the start of the week. I needed to take a different approach and control the controllables.

I started going to bed earlier, at a consistent time: between 09:00 p.m. and 10:00 p.m. With enough sleep, that was one less excuse. I even bought caffeine tablets to place on my bedside drawer. I didn't drink coffee at the time, but it seemed like a smart trick to play on myself. The alarm would blast, and I'd whack a 200mg caffeine tablet (equivalent to an espresso) down my gullet before I knew my arse from my elbow. *Well, you ain't gettin' back to sleep now sonny boy, up and at 'em.* Another change I made was to make the transition from bed to the pavement as quick and painless as possible. To remove time for thinking from the equation when I would make an excuse to go back to bed, I laid out all my running essentials the night before, placing them at the foot of my bed. From that point on, there was much less friction, but boy did I find the bed to footpath process hard to conquer at first.

It's not safe to rely on being super motivated every single day. That's why I needed these tricks. Some days I was like a dog biting and pulling on his leash, jumping out of bed, raring to go. There were many more days I wanted nothing more than the comfort and security of my blanket. When motivation lacked, discipline *had* to kick in. Luckily, I'd learned the habits of discipline from my sporting youth and just needed to drill it back in place. Nevermind fluctuating motivation, without discipline I knew I would fail.

No matter how begrudgingly I might have left the cosiness of the indoors and exposed myself to the elements, I never recalled any time where I returned thinking, *I wish I didn't go training.* There was always at least a small sense of accomplishment from conquering the lazy voice in my head, moving, being outdoors, and from the endorphins flowing through my body afterwards. I needed to remind myself of this if I hesitated about training – and even say it aloud if required.

Come January 2012, I'd started the official training plan. I was already struggling with my increasingly demanding schedule – longer, more frequent runs, lectures, assignment due dates looming and getting the bus home from Dublin to work in Waterford. With the trajectory of the weekly distances only going up, my time management had to become military. I couldn't afford to let any of the spinning plates drop.

After the months of socialising like a good thing, as a regular student, I was firmly back on the straight and narrow and saying no. *No, I can't go slugging pints. No, I can't go to the cinema.* I was already spread thinly and needed to prioritise. I needed to go without some pleasures for a little while, and I was okay with that. I was focused on the mission and knew I couldn't half-arse it. It didn't feel like a sacrifice at the time, more a logical and necessary step if I wanted to succeed.

SHOW UP

The Heart Foundation's Corporate Fundraising Manager invited me to join her at a runner's clinic, along with the charity's Activity

Events Manager. They wanted me to speak, plug my fundraiser run and entice others to fundraise for their charity. 53 Degrees North hosted the evening in their Carrickmines store, and the charity thought those guys might sponsor me for the essential gear if I did it. I literally couldn't afford to say no and was happy to give up half my day to do my bit in our quest for sponsors. I hadn't a clue what to be saying to the attendees, though. I wasn't a good salesman. In my eyes, I hadn't done a tap worth discussing and felt like a right imposter. Who was I to be standing up and telling a group of experienced middle-aged distance runners what I was planning to do? *Some cheek this fecker!*

'How many marathons have you completed so far, do you mind me asking?' came the first question after my short spiel.

'Just done Dublin last October.'

'Wow, only one? What time did you do it in, out of interest?'

'Eh, about 4 hours and 10 minutes.'

They did not look impressed or convinced. I couldn't blame the audience in the slightest. I had run my first ever marathon in an average time just two months before that and claimed I would run 35 back-to-back marathons in about five months. It's safe to say I died on my arse during my presentation, but I got the clothing sponsorship I was after: North Face shorts and sun cap, compression socks, Under Armour t-shirts and most importantly, six pairs of runners. It just proves that it's often just about showing up and giving things an honest bash. I was scared, nervous and felt I had no right to be speaking, but saying yes to the opportunity paid off and saved a grand or two in expenses. Not being afraid to fall can be a dangerous character trait, but it can come in handy at times!

MOMENTUM

Up until February, I was riding the growing wave of momentum. On the running side of things, I went from zero to running the Dublin Marathon and realising how deluded I was. Then, I went back to the drawing board, approaching things correctly, following structured training, day in, day out. Days of commitment soon layered to weeks, which became months. Now, I was able to run 130 kilometres in a week, including solitary training marathons before college. My classmates were still snoring, some just getting home from a house session, and I'd run 42 kilometres. *Oorah*!

At this point in my development, a week could look like this:

Monday – 13 kilometres

Tuesday – 10 kilometres

Wednesday – 42 kilometres

Thursday – 8 kilometres

Friday – 16 kilometres

Saturday – 8 kilometres

Sunday – 32 kilometres

I wasn't running these at a blistering pace. The focus was consistency, not intensity: time on the feet, slow, building extreme endurance capabilities, whilst avoiding overexertion, injury and resulting forced time off. There were no medals, money, or cheers, just the satisfaction in achieving a silent solo training marathon and getting another step closer to the goal.

I felt I had come a *long* way in a short space of time. Running the October Marathon with no foundation and experiencing the wheels falling off the bus was a world apart from now. Resetting and laying a solid foundation, a brick at a time, doing 10–20% more volume each week. I couldn't stop to admire my half-finished piece of work, though. *You ran marathons before class – so what! You're a long way from the real goal. Keep the head down.* There were sores and niggles for sure, but the kilometres were gradually accumulating.

Aside from the running momentum, other aspects of the project were gaining momentum too, like convincing myself to commit, telling Gerry – a stranger – and then my dad, followed by the rest of my family and friends. The website and online donation link were live, thanks to the charity. There was no hiding place now. There was some traction in the community too, with people now donating money towards the causes. I felt right on track. I was holding up my end of the bargain, looking after my physical preparation and study commitments, whilst also going above and beyond, off my own bat, unlocking some donation money for the charities.

Another momentous milestone was doing the press launch. Dad managed to convince Giovanni Trapattoni to help with the publicity. Giovanni Trapattoni was the Irish football team manager at the time. He had hundreds of appearances for AC Milan as a player. His managerial career is second to none, managing the likes of AC Milan, Juventus, Inter Milan, Bayern Munich, and Italy. It was an absolute honour having such a prestigious sportsman give his stamp of approval and lend his profile to my event and its causes. He was down in Waterford for some media obligations anyway, so he didn't mind being pulled aside for a quick photo or two and wished me the best of luck. What a gentleman!

The photos were a bit cheesy: me, in my shorts and charity t-shirt, in between my dad holding a heart-shaped prop and Giovanni in his tailored Italian suit. The images served their purpose and appeared in the national papers. The charity's 'Marathon Man' PR hook worked a treat, newspapers regurgitating the phrase in headlines, as the subheading declared 'Alan Corcoran will be running 35 marathons in 35 days around Ireland, in aid of charity'. Whatever the chances of doing a U-turn up to that point, appearing in national print and online media with the donation link meant the exit door was now firmly shut.

The project was picking up steam. It was an exciting time, upping the kilometres, as more people became aware of my efforts and started donating.

FIVE:

STUBBORN PERSISTENCE

HURDLES

The positivity bubble I was growing got stabbed with a pin at the end of February 2012, when the Heart Foundation contacted me.

'I think we should meet up this week, if possible? I'm getting concerned with the lack of reaction we've got from potential sponsors, and I think we should sit down and go through it all. I'm particularly worried about the logistics operation.'

For fuck sake, I thought. *I'm a final year college student, just turned 21, busting my balls off to hold up my end of the bargain, now officially doing crazy training, studying and working like goodo; pulling in cash donations to boot. I don't have time or energy to meet with the professional to discuss his difficulties with the logistics that he'd volunteered to take care of.* I don't imagine he'd have been overly enamoured by me if he'd secured sponsors, and I requested a meeting to discuss how hard my running training was and how little I had completed. We were five months on from our handshake and only three months out from the start of the run. Meeting to talk with me about it seemed to waste time when he could be proactively solving problems. *Just do what you said you would,* was the frustrated and simplistic response in my head. We were a team, so I had to take a deep breath, be patient and polite and hear him out.

Having completed my 32-kilometre training jog for the morning, I hopped onto the Luas and headed to Dublin City's Italian Quarter. I queued up and ordered my cup of tea while giving a smile and wave to the sharply dressed fundraising professional, already punctually sitting in his chair. I sat down across the table, feeling very underdressed in my hoody and tracksuit bottoms; swinging my backpack to rest by my mud-speckled trainers.

The gist of the meeting was that the charity hadn't organised much. They'd launched the website, emailed a press statement around and secured the opportunity for me to talk at the 53 Degrees North store, leading to the store sponsoring some running attire.

The charity's representative was now putting their hands up, in March, confessing to underestimating the work involved. The charity's original thinking was to call a handful of targeted multinationals and get large cash sponsors upfront – quick win and profits generated. That was plan A. However, they couldn't find easy cash sponsors willing to contribute and cover expenses. According to them, their plan B of calling hotels didn't work either. None were willing to provide any accommodation or food for my team and me. Nor was there a single physio in place or a support vehicle sourced. The elements the charity had offered to take responsibility for looked in dire shape.

Having told him about Gerry and Ken's success in raising €500,000, I got the impression the charity had high hopes – as did I – thinking it would be simple and straightforward to get lucrative support from big business and the public. After all, I was embarking on an unusual endurance challenge that surpassed Gerry and Ken by an extra 126.2 kilometres. My event was unique, in that I would be the first person to run a lap of Ireland. My challenge also had more of an emotive angle, given it was kickstarted by the impact of my dad's stroke. Dad had a public profile, too, from his years of work for the Football Association. When it all started, there seemed to be plenty of hooks to effortlessly reel in sponsors and media, generating charity donations. I had broadly the same ingredients as Eddie, Terry, Dean, Gerry and Ken. The Heart Foundation, my family, my friends and I shared the same optimistic feeling at first. It seemed to be a winning formula.

Beyond thinking it should be handy to secure sponsors and generate donations, I hadn't given it further consideration, primarily because the professionals had told me to leave it to them. With months faded by, they were now dragging me back to the table to ponder the dilemma with them.

'Look, I know this sounds awful, Alan, but being blunt, there's nothing wrong with you. You're a normal healthy young male student running marathons, which is fantastic, of course, but you're not blind, or on one leg, so we're having a hard time convincing companies to part with their cash.'

I nearly spat my tea out. The statement jarred me for

a second, but that was the reality. As impressive a feat or as marketable as my run may seem to us, I was not a Terry Fox. I was not a cancer patient with an amputated leg. Nor was I a celebrity, like Eddie Izzard. It was still strange to hear it from the charity's mouth, but I couldn't argue with facts. I appreciated the honesty, albeit a bit late. Business is business, and the media are the media. They want something sensational to attract eyeballs and profit. What I was doing was not edgy enough or pulling on enough heartstrings for corporates, judging by the Heart Foundation's words and their fruitless attempts at securing the necessary pieces of the logistics puzzle.

The charity had only just researched Gerry and Ken's success, which was too little too late in my view. As I've touched on, those head-the-ball runners generated hype and donations by inviting individuals to run an organised marathon or half-marathon in each of the 32 counties they ran in. My challenge didn't have that component by design. My challenge differed in its more straightforward format without any bells and whistles, or crowds. I was planning to head off on the open road, with two friends in a support car, and run the most scenic routes home via the Irish coastline. That was the dream. If people wanted to join informally, they could – the more the merrier – but I didn't have the desire or resources to organise ratified events with participants and safety protocols on each of the 35 days.

With the charity eventually speaking to Gerry, they were now fixating on altering the terms of our agreement. The fundraiser told me they were now 'very determined' for me to run the official Waterford Viking Marathon route. The alteration in the challenge would allow the charity to encourage people to 'run with Alan', creating a half-arsed version of Gerry and Ken's successful participatory method of fundraising.

I'm thinking, *This is March, lads, and I'm starting in May, for God's sake. You can't seriously want me to change the challenge format now?* I was floored by the request to reroute at this late stage of the game. I had been chipping away for months at the crack of dawn, consistently doing what I said I would do. The charity publicly advertised me in the national press to run 35 marathons in 35 days, a lap of Ireland, on their behalf. They were now pressuring me into one of two alternatives:

1 – Almost run a lap of Ireland, stopping one marathon short of a complete lap and driving to Waterford to partake in the Waterford Viking Marathon, the 35th marathon on the 35th day.

2 – Run a lap of Ireland, 35 marathons in 35 days, as agreed and advertised, but run an additional 36th marathon on the 36th day, the Waterford Viking Marathon.

Option one wasn't a runner for me. I said no immediately. My ambition and commitment to everyone since the start was to run a lap of Ireland. This option was not a lap of Ireland, and I wasn't willing to cut the gigantic loop short by 42.2 kilometres, to drive the last 2.8% home. No way, Jose.

Option two made me bite my tongue instead of saying, *Cheeky fucker! Are you taking the piss?* To me, this option was even more disrespectful than Option one. Again, I said no, as this wasn't what we agreed on in September. I was fuming inside but kept a neutral outward appearance. I felt my extreme efforts and the enormity of the challenge were hugely underappreciated. There seemed to be a disconnect with the reality of what extra lengths they were asking of me; flippant about wanting me to run another 42.2 kilometres at the end of doing so for five weeks straight.

'I can't do either, sorry. That's not what we agreed and not what I told everyone I would be doing. You even issued a press release, declaring: "Marathon Man: Lap of Ireland Run, 35 Marathons in 35 Days". It's in black and white headlines now. These options don't match our advert. I sent you my route back in November, detailing every single stage of the run. Couldn't you just organise a participatory marathon on any number of those 35 routes if you want to entice people to run with me and chip in money? That way, I'm sticking to my guns, and you've got the "run with Alan" PR spin to try to sell?'

'Unfortunately, we don't have the time or resources to pull that off at this stage, and the Viking Marathon is ready-made, with no costs for us,' was the rebuttal.

I felt frustrated, let down and isolated. The lack of completed tasks on their side and insistence on changing tack stung.

Despite my general inexperience, I was glad I stuck to my values. It was intimidating. I was this unqualified student, and he was a senior professional representing a national charity, leaning heavily on me to fold. I didn't think it was right to break my promises or be made run an extra marathon. It was no skin off their nose, but I was the face and voice of my fundraiser challenge, and it meant everything for me to do what I visualised and said I would, as painfully stubborn as I may have come across to them. I went to the charity with a proposal and possibilities for them to try to make the most of. I didn't feel I needed to compromise on my dream, commitments and character because of the charity's difficulties in exploiting the opportunity I gave them.

Undeterred by my steadfast attitude during the meeting, the charity continued to push for me to concede to them. In steps, my dad to the rescue. We had to arrange yet another meeting, the three of us this time. Boy, was I thankful my father had made such an impressive return from his stroke! It meant the world to me to have him by my side to mediate.

We sat down in a hotel lobby over a pot of tea, and I started by setting out my stall. My dad understood I wanted to run a lap of Ireland, completing 35 marathons in 35 days, as agreed. The fundraiser said his piece and my dad understood he wanted me to run the Viking Marathon as an opportunity to boost the fundraising aspect. We were both too focused on our juxtaposed positions. Football administration, conflict resolution and chairing boardroom meetings was my dad's forte. Dad chimed in effortlessly.

'What about an alternative? Just a suggestion: could you revise the route, Al? It would still be a lap of Ireland, just a tighter circle, adjusting the 35 stages to squeeze 42.2 kilometres out of the loop. That way, you'd still run the lap of Ireland, just as 34 marathons in 34 days, and you could then do the Viking Marathon as a victory lap of sorts – the 35th marathon on the 35th day? Although different, it keeps you true to your word – a lap of Ireland and 35 consecutive marathons. It means you're not doing 36 marathons, *definitely not*. That tweak seems like you can both get what you want? A win-win?'

I must say, I was impressed by my dad's quick, measured and clear-sighted input. I was committed to my vision, but I allowed some flexibility in my approach with encouragement from Dad. I think the fundraiser and I both felt like eejits not seeing that solution. We could both live with that.

Simple as that! With the agreement to revise the route, we moved to the remaining problems. During our correspondences, I had questioned what the fundraiser has done to secure accommodation over the last five months. I didn't get an answer. It seemed peculiar to me that no hotel or restaurant would be willing to get involved and help. During the meeting, it transpired that the charity had contacted three big chain hotels, but they weren't interested. This was enough for them to conclude, *We can't get accommodation*. To me, this would be a sign to use common sense, accept the easiest option didn't work and change the angle of attack. Move on to ring local hotels near each day's finish line. Local hotels were the more practical solution anyhow. Pinballing between a large chain hotel in a city and each day's rural finish line was impractical, losing hours each day to an unnecessary commute. It seemed they chose the path of least effort over the best approach. With Dad's presence, I at least had the answer, and now knew why we had no accommodation or food yet. It didn't instil any confidence. I wanted to just put my head in my hands there and then. I felt I was committed to them and my promise.

At that moment, it didn't feel like they were committed to me or their promise. *Why am I bothering putting myself through all this to raise money for their cause, if they can't be arsed with their end of the bargain? They volunteered to cover it. What have they been up to all these months?* I was reassured to know it wasn't just me having major doubts; my dad left the meeting unimpressed with the response regarding food and accommodation and their insistence on the late change to our terms of the agreement.

Jesus, was I delighted for Dad's presence and useful input! He could see that it was a great unnecessary stress off my shoulders to have that crap sorted. I could see he felt useful, adding value to the project; helping me out of a bind. There was satisfaction for us in our teamwork at least.

With a line under the route and the 'run with Alan' problem, I spent a day in the college library painstakingly re-doing my stack of digital maps. Losing the 35th marathon stage to the Viking Marathon loop, meant significant adjustments were needed. After meticulously adjusting the routes, I sent the revised plans to the Heart Foundation, in the hope they would stay true to their word.

While all the logistics nonsense was going on, I was sucking diesel on the trails. I was in the middle of a bonkers training block – a 120-kilometre week, followed by a 137-kilometre week, followed by a 145-kilometre week. To reach these distances, I was predominantly running around 16 kilometres per day. That was now my bread and butter. I was contrasting the standard runs, with one or two long runs per week at that point. *Long,* as in up to 50-kilometres long, having done a 32-kilometre training run days prior.

My body was undoubtedly tired, the drain on my spirits from the organisational side taking an added toll. At the end of the tunnel of this intense block of work, I had some light – the relief of *only* having a 65-kilometre week. What had been a testing week a few months before was now called my easy recovery week. There were no crowds like the Dublin Marathon to encourage me through tough times and no medals to strive for. Still, the buzz of completing solitary 50-kilometre runs gave me enough positive feedback to keep persevering, despite the hurdles coming out of left field.

Bar my roommates and immediate family, nobody knew the extent of the time I was putting in on the roads. That said, my barber, Danny, noticed and complimented my commitment, having spotted me running into the small hours, a few weekends on the trot, as he was getting a taxi from the local pub to the city nightclub! I felt like a maverick pounding the pavement on a Friday and Saturday night, my friends all out clubbing. After sweating in my kitchen scrubs at work, I'd start pounding the pavement. It was an acceptable price to pay for my newly accumulated power of being able to head off under my own steam for hours on end. I was happy to temporarily forgo the immediate fun and pleasure of youth, for achievement and long-term self-esteem.

CAN'T WALK

Siobhan Fitzpatrick was a chartered physio in Waterford Regional Hospital, ran her own private practice and was the Waterford Senior Hurling team's physio too. She was from the same neck of the woods as me, with a sprinting background as well. Despite her manic schedule, Siobhan was generous enough to make time to look after my aches and pains for the months of training. When she wasn't available, she roped in her colleague, Rory Carthy, and even linked me up with Roy Brennan, a great Physical Therapist who could patch me up when I was in Dublin.

Off the back of my biggest training block to date, where I climbed to 145 kilometres in a week, came a critical recovery week. I thought it was sensible timing to pop to the physio to relieve some of my aches. Relief, wasn't what I got, however. At least not in the short term. My calves were obviously a little tight and my knees a tad tender; given the mileage I was putting on them. Luckily, I didn't have any drastic injuries and no real troubling niggles. I told Rory as much before he had a poke around to feel for himself.

'Oh, that does feel rough now. Yep, ow, fuck!' was my revised assessment, as Rory jabbed his hardened physio thumb into my calves.

'Want me to ease off?'

'No, not at all. It's a rest week with a full day off tomorrow. Do what ya gotta do. I can hack it.'

We were in the middle of the concrete dressing room in Walsh Park, before a Waterford hurling match. I was there early, so as not to disrupt the team's match preparations. As the torture was commencing, a few friends from my school days strolled in, Stephen O'Keefe, Barry Coughlan, Philip and Pauric Mahony. They laughed at my wincing face as they patted me on the back, knowing all too well the joys of getting a sports massage on heavily used muscles. I thought Rory's squeezing thumb was terrible at first, but that was pleasant compared to what was next.

'You have a full day off tomorrow, you said? A low mileage week for the rest of this week, until starting into your next climb?'

'That sounds like a loaded question but spot on.'

'Okay for me to do some dry needling?'

'I haven't a clue what that is, but I'll trust ya. Fire away.'

Rory felt for one of the many tight knots and sore points in my now scrawny distance runner legs, then, he stuck a needle into the muscle and moved it around a bit. If he got the right spot, the muscle would start twitching uncontrollably, as an intense pain surged. It's such a strange sensation. I've got a high tolerance for pain but, Japers Jack, this was next level! Every needle Rory inserted felt worse than the last, as my calf muscles danced like someone trying to escape a straitjacket.

'Is that normal?' I could just about ask, as I squeezed the sides of the cushioned physio table. The agony was my just desserts for laughing at poor Eddie Izzard squirm on TV all those years ago.

'Eh, I've never seen it this bad, no. Normally you get a twitch here and there, but every needle is twitching like crazy. Is it too much for you?'

'It is but keep stabbing. I want to be tip-top for the next block.'

The dry needling was meant to stimulate the muscles to repair quicker, increasing the blood flow to the area which needed healing. I didn't want to deter him going as hard as he felt necessary, so I stuck a towel over my grimacing face and shut up, focusing on breathing and absorbing the punishment he was dishing out. I mean 'treatment', sorry!

I was a beginner distance runner, covering distances on the brink of, and likely beyond, the verge of stupid, upping the volume about 20% each week. My muscles were tighter than most and the associated twitching and pain greater than most too. With my face hidden, so the pain wasn't visible, Rory didn't hold back as I continued to brace myself. It was kind of like the response when you stub your toe on the kitchen table, but way worse because it kept getting stubbed every 20 seconds.

'Ah, fucker, huh, phoo, breathe! Ah, shit, phoo …!'

I thanked Siobhan and Rory, wished the lads the best of luck in their game and walked out to my mother, who was waiting in her car outside the stadium to collect me.

Fifteen minutes later, I was home. The drive was enough time for both my calves to have seized up after the treatment. I could barely walk as I attempted to get from the driveway to the front door. It reminded me of having a sprained ankle. You might play on or walk for a bit after the initial twist, but once cooled down, it stiffens like an iron poker, and the pain intensifies significantly. I appreciate that analogy might only translate to the minority foolhardy as me, stupid enough to try to plough on despite a sprained ankle.

My mam was not best pleased with the state of me, shuffling to the front door. Her fears of her youngest son damaging himself were now evident as I limped to the couch for some sweet stationary respite.

Around an hour later, I needed to pee. The additional time

meant my legs felt even worse than before. It was easier, faster and less painful to take my legs out of the equation. Looking like Leonardo DiCaprio crawling towards his Lamborghini on Quaaludes in *The Wolf of Wall Street*, I dragged my limp legs slowly behind me on my elbows, heading for the bathroom. I felt eyes on me as I crawled from the sitting room. I looked right, from the hallway floor and into the kitchen. Who was standing there looking down on me? Only my mother, shaking her head in utter disappointment.

'Ah Alan!'

'What?' I laughed as if there was nothing to see here.

Mam pulled an old pair of crutches out of the garage, so I could get the bus back to college that evening as planned. I asked my roommate, Simon, to meet me off the bus to help carry my bags to our flat. I was barely capable of holding myself up, never mind bags.

'Well boy, what the fuck happened to you?' Simon asked.

'Ah, I just went to the physio.'

'Aren't you meant to hobble into the physio and leave the place in better shape? Not walk in without a bother and hobble out?'

He raised a fair point, but I trusted Rory, who had said I'd feel sore for a day but should be good as new come tomorrow. I didn't have much choice but to hope and wait. I certainly hadn't anticipated feeling this beat up, and it was hard to see me going from crutches to running freely after one night's sleep. The next day I wasn't in shape to run, but I was walking without too much restriction. Come the following day; I was back on the trails for 16 kilometres. I felt fantastic. It worked. I was equal parts impressed and surprised by the process. My calves and knees were spick-and-span, despite the suffering I had to endure to get them to feel that way. I rang my mother to reassure her I was back flying it, much to her relief.

'I just don't want you hurting yourself,' she repeated for the thousandth time.

'It'll be grand, Mam.'

This recovery week experience re-emphasised the stress my body was and would be under, and the importance physios could play in the success or failure of getting me to the start line and then to the finish line. I was around eight weeks out from the start of the challenge. To my frustration, the charity hadn't secured one physio along the route yet. Like contacting the big hotel chains, getting a no and being satisfied in the fruitless outcome, they approached the physio task in the same manner. Contacting the Irish Society of Chartered Physiotherapists, they got no response and advised me to 'forget it at this stage.' They had a contact who put them onto someone else, who put them onto a third person, who apparently couldn't give an answer. This conclusion was the result of six months' work. *Great help*, I thought. I was left high and dry on yet another item they had volunteered to take responsibility for. I was fuming. Because the overarching physio body had ignored them, they seemed content to give up. The sourcing of zero physios was another real blow to morale when I questioned why I was still bothering with my end of the deal.

With no physios secured, I had no choice but to give up

on pointlessly chasing the charity for results and had to try and progress this aspect myself. My physio, Siobhan Fitzpatrick, was the superwoman to the rescue. She was part counsellor too, by now, listening to my operational gripes as I carried out her stretching instructions. She was as annoyed as me at the situation, seeing first-hand the stress I was putting my body through. Her phrase was, 'If you want something done, ask a busy person.' More than words, she took it upon herself to help and started reaching out to physios along my planned route. Siobhan's attitude alone was enough to restore my faith in people and pick me up.

Since my challenge had the advantage of knowing exactly where I'd be each day and roughly what time, we could be quite detailed and focused on the hunt for and pitch to local physios. Armed with the relative certainty of places and dates, we found physios were more than willing to help the challenge, gladly contributing 30-60 minutes of their time. With Siobhan's help, there was a handful of physios in the spreadsheet within mere days. The confirmations made me so happy, knowing I'd have treatment on the route. I also got a competitive sense of satisfaction. The professional said to forget finding physios after having months to source them. Among her many commitments, Siobhan was single-handedly making decent inroads, in a fraction of the time. It begged the question, did the charity try much at all? I was having my doubts. Maybe we just had different definitions of what trying meant and had different concepts of what taking responsibility for something should entail.

TALKING SHITE

There were hundreds of kilometres still to run in training, edging towards the peak in volume, and logistics responsibilities were taking up more of my time than anticipated. I was getting to the business end of my college degree too, with final assignments coming due, right at the wrong time. Despite feeling like I was already being pulled from pillar to post, further responsibilities were being added to my plate. The distractions came in the form of media requests shortly after the charity issued the press release.

I initially thought the paid charity employees would be the salespeople and cheerleaders putting in the energy and doing the plugging – the promotor if you will. It didn't work like that. Journalists wanted to speak with the source. Most print and online media wanted a unique direct quote, rather than merely copying and pasting from the sheet of A4 shared by the charity. The press release wasn't much good for radio or TV unless I showed up and talked shite when requests for my time were made. It fell on my shoulders to answer the calls.

I hadn't given much thought to this additional voluntary duty initially. It was a charity running adventure I signed up for, not a charity talkathon. I didn't feel the desire or need to try to verbally justify and sell my challenge. *Can I not just run a lap of Ireland, no?*

I'm a firm believer that talk is cheap and actions speak louder than words, and that's what the challenge was about, taking action. Rightly or wrongly, that's not the real world. The reality of it sucked a bit. If I talked a game as well as Conor McGregor, but I didn't back it up by completing the run, I could conceivably raise way more for charity than if I successfully ran in silence. I could run up Everest blindfolded and backwards, but if I didn't do promotional work and only my family and close friends knew about it, there would be shag-all donations to show for it at the end of the day. Organic word of mouth wouldn't generate many donations unless I had rich friends. I don't. That's one lesson I had to get my head around.

I had to change my attitude if I was serious about raising as much money for the charities as possible. Although this desire was waning with my recent exchanges with the charity, I was still deadly serious. I knew the fundraising meant a lot for Dad too. He knew first-hand what the money could do for the Football Village of Hope and wanted to repay the NRH for their efforts during his recovery.

As an inexperienced student, it was a new and exciting challenge to go to a radio studio or TV station to be questioned for the first time – a character-building experience. My trial by fire was going live with Ivan Yates and Chris Donoghue on *Newstalk Breakfast*, and then there was *Craig Doyle Live* on TV, with Jason McAteer and Jason Byrne. The schedule was too much, and this aspect of volunteering quickly became a chore. Marketing is not a strength of mine, and it was an uncomfortable task dealing with repetitive leading questions after leading questions from journalists about a challenging life experience.

'Would you say your Dad has always been a loving father? He took you to football practice as a child. Isn't that right? It must have been very hard living away from home when your Dad suffered a severe stroke, wasn't it?' If unsuccessful in their first attempt, they'd ask the same question in a slightly different way until I gave them the quote they were trying to spoon-feed me. It was nerve-wracking putting myself on the spot, under the magnifying glass of public scrutiny. Imagine doing a job interview in an area you began studying a few months prior. You have to sound intelligent, sincere, funny, and of course, yourself, while needing to blow your own trumpet to sell the gravity of the undertaking but not too hard because nobody likes a big head. Now imagine there's an audience of hundreds or thousands watching or listening live, and judging – awful stuff altogether.

There was an expectation to do this unpaid extra work all the same. The charity hadn't got the sponsors they initially thought they'd get, so I'd be sent in to ask on-air for sponsors and direct the public to the online donation link to get money into the charity's coffers. Despite feeling short-changed by being the only person in the equation not getting paid, I had to ask myself if I wanted to run, or if I wanted to run and fundraise for a more significant cause beyond personal adventure. I concluded I'd just say yes to doing free media work and stop wrestling with the idea of it being an unwanted burden. It would be for the charity's benefit and give me more satisfaction with a more respectable fundraising bottom line to show. The greater the pot of gold for the charities at the end, the more impressed and prouder my family would be too. So, talk, I did.

It was all an education nonetheless – some more eye-opening real-world experience. I learned it's best not to listen back to interviews. *You sound like a gobshite!* It prepared me for graduate job interviews and fielding questions. It also prepared me for discovering my time had no monetary value yet in the real world, interning unpaid for months, hoping that my college degree would someday entitle me to at least the minimum wage for an honest day's work.

BACK-TO-BACK

Another recovery week behind me and a massive test on the first week of the next three-week building block. This was the 'hell block'. It was time to try back-to-back marathons in training. *Oh boy*. Saturday: a solo marathon in the Phoenix Park, comfortably hitting 4 hours and 30 minutes, ice bin (I had no bath), eat, rehydrate, rest, sleep. Sunday: same again, hitting 4 hours and 30 minutes on the nose like clockwork. Mentally, this was a monumental weekend where I proved to myself that I'd come on leaps and bounds since the Dublin Marathon in October. I was a different animal entirely. It instilled confidence: confidence I had earned through hard work and repetition.

The 80+ kilometres over two days also felt as if it was nothing. Nobody knew what I was up to. I looked like a normal – albeit slow – jogger, just out for a potter in the park. There were no celebrations or accolades to be had. I just showered and hit the library to work on my final year assignments for the rest of my Sunday. As strange as it sounds, it just felt normal. Because of my consistent training, my body absorbed the runs like I had only done an hour walk on the beach on Saturday and an hour walk on the beach on Sunday. The body can be moulded into phenomenal shape if your mind is willing to put in the hours of steady graft.

THE WALL

I learned 'the wall' is real and never wanted to experience it again. I was confident in my endurance ability come early April, having ticked over the 32-kilometre mark more than 10 times by then. All the more reason why this wobbly experience took me by surprise and stuck out in my mind.

Reducing my time from bed to pavement to make sure I started running, meant no sitting around eating breakfast and wasting time letting the food settle. If the run would be less than an hour, I'd neck a glass of water and head off. If I was out for more than an hour, I'd have my CamelBak hydration backpack and wore compression sleeves with food stashed up them. I might stash a homemade gel or cereal bar and just carry a banana to have on the go. It depended on how far I was planning to run.

In a rush to get moving and now confident in my endurance abilities, on this early morning's 26-kilometre run around the Phoenix Park, I packed much lighter than usual on the food front. To compound matters, I hadn't refuelled as much as I should have after my previous evening's run.

Everything was typical and comfortable until about kilometre 19, but then I started feeling strangely lethargic. Something wasn't right. I decided to take a shortcut to try to get to the exit of the park and home sooner than scheduled. Although my body felt like it was shutting down, my mind said, *Don't be a lazy quitter; struggle through.* When I reached the exit, I forced myself back into the park to ensure I would get the planned distance covered.

It was around 09:00 a.m., and the suits were moving into

the nearby Criminal Courts of Justice and the city centre. I, on the other hand, was dishevelled, no longer capable of a straight line. This morning's run was much more concerning than the Dublin Marathon's midway point, when I was sorer and more tired than I felt I should be, self-doubts kicking in with a daunting distance ahead. This training run was utter exhaustion, with my body getting more and more unresponsive. *Why is this happening after just 19 kilometres of only 26 kilometres?* I was thinking.

I had slowed dramatically and was veering off course, struggling to correct myself. I 'ran', if you can call it that, deep enough back into the park to know I'd hit the training distance, provided I lived long enough to make it back to my flat. I had my doubts. I had an urge like never before to stop, lie down and call for help. Hunched over, hands on my knees, I was cursing myself. *Aw, you twat, why did you go further from home?* My engine felt empty, and I was not well at all. This intense state felt like a full-on survival mode. *You have to make it home, Al. Just a step at a time. Sitting or stopping is only going to prolong the suffering. Get home!* On the brink of what felt like collapse and looking like a sleep-deprived drunk with an athletic fashion sense, I stumbled in slow zig-zags towards my Stoneybatter flat.

The contrast of my state to the surrounding environment was comical in hindsight, although I didn't much appreciate it at the time. Sweat-soaked, with my empty Dora the Explorer hydration pack, I was a right mess, staggering past groomed professionals with metallic coffee mugs in hand and silent concern etched on their faces. Even the criminals smoking on the court's steps looked at me with pity and gave me space as I apologetically took the most direct line of travel to the next turn in the road.

It took me about a year to get from the park's gate, along Arbour Hill, to my flat, just 1.2 kilometres away, pausing every few shuffles to rest my hand on the old red terraced brickwork.

Once home, I slumped on the kitchen floor, feeling fit for A&E. I limply dragged out anything that contained sugar and was within arm's reach from the cupboard and onto the floor. Like Father Ted's Sister Assumpta, during Lent, I horsed the chocolates into me. Supported by the walls either side, I dragged my sorry ass down the hall to the shower room and sat under the therapeutic flow of warm water, waiting for the sugar to hit me like a drug and hoping it would solve all my problems.

After about 15 minutes, I was a new man. *That was nuts, but at least you didn't shit your shorts, good man,* was my thought as I headed out the door for a full day of college. From that point on, I made sure to have more food on me than I planned to consume – 'tear wrapper in case of emergency'. If I was doing an evening or night run followed by a morning run, I ensured I dialled in my nutrition more too. I now knew the results of underdoing it and never wanted to feel in that zombie state ever again: live and learn!

TEAMWORK

The distances and dates were regimented. If I didn't make it to the day's finish line in time, i.e. within 24 hours, I would be ending the challenge in failure. I wasn't going to move the goalposts mid-challenge. This made the organising somewhat uncomplicated, compared to mountain-based or sea-based endurance events, which are dictated by Mother Nature, an all-powerful variable that ensures you can't confidently plan anything beyond a day at a time. The run was simple. Come hail, rain or shine, I'd move my ass 42.2 kilometres further along the road with each passing day. The fixed nature of the schedule made sourcing a team that bit easier. It was quite an unskilled role in support, making this Irish journey an accessible beast. Being road-based meant they wouldn't require a folder of survival qualifications, essential on many off-road adventures. The only prerequisite was that at least one of the two team members was licenced to drive.

The job of sourcing a support team was made much simpler by my good childhood friend and neighbour Tom Davies, taking annual leave and unpaid leave from his PWC accountancy job. He committed to help me with three of the five weeks. He was a safe and reliable pair of hands and ensured continuity for a large chunk of the challenge, minimising the need for repeated team inductions, which was fantastic news. I was young, and so were my friends, mostly just finishing college, footloose without kids and mortgages restricting us. As a result, I filled in all the team slots with relative ease and plenty of spare time.

WHEELS IN MOTION

Noticing the trajectory of the organising side of things and realising there was still no support vehicle, I decided to play it safe and focus my attention on quietly going after an event car sponsor myself. The vehicle cover was a significant concern up until then. *Will I have to run on my own? How will I carry all my gear, food and liquids? How will I get to my accommodation and physio appointments after each marathon?*

Thankfully, my efforts paid off pretty quickly with one connection coming good. A parent of two girls I went to primary school with stepped up. John Flood's Dungarvan Nissan dealership in Waterford offered me a vehicle loan for the challenge's duration. Securing the car loan was a mammoth win. I'd spent time pleading with friends and family to slot into my excel spreadsheet, giving up their time for free, ensuring I had a two-person support team at all times for the five weeks. Most didn't own a car yet, so I badly needed one. Securing it meant my team just needed to bring themselves and their driver's licence, and we were good to go. With a support car guaranteed, I no longer had to consider messy alternatives.

ULTRA-RUNNING

I had piled up a fair few accomplishments in training by now: a handful of 32-kilometre runs, some 42.2-kilometre marathons and back-to-back marathons. The 3rd April 2012, saw me hit my training peak: over 185 kilometres in a single week. It also saw me complete my longest individual run too. I was pencilled to do a 50-kilometre training run. The logic was that, although I'd be running 42.2 kilometres, day in and day out on the challenge, I needed to be confident that I could run longer and spend more time on my feet if needs be. With my back-to-back training marathons completed, I was hoping the 35 consecutive marathons would continue on that path of consistent 4-hour and 30-minute marathons. If injury struck though, my marathon training times would be unlikely. These long slow 50-kilometre sessions would prepare me physically and mentally for that eventuality.

Although I loved running on the Phoenix Park's trails, a sanctuary from the harsher road running, I hadn't run with anyone since October's Dublin Marathon. I saw the Connemarathon ultramarathon broadly coincided with my scheduled 50-kilometre training run. I thought it would make a refreshing change of scenery: something different to break the monotony and test myself. *Feck it, why not that 64-kilometre race instead?* What're a few extra kilometres? It would be nice to run with people for a change and trial my newly received runners, sponsored by 53 Degrees North.

My Dad and I set off to Connemara. It was lovely to get away for a weekend together. It was great that he had regained the freedom and ability to drive there, without a bother. I met Gerry Duffy there selling his book at the race registration event and updated him on my steady progress. He was delighted for me, which is a sign of the man he is, encouraging others to succeed. I thanked him profusely for his instrumental help in getting me to where I was and left him to drum up some book business. While most runners had been sensibly tapering down, easing off on their distances before the ultra, I was at the end of my biggest week yet. I had even run 24 kilometres the previous day.

The uninhabited wild scenery was spectacular. You couldn't help but smile in the secluded postcard setting of lakes, mountains, sheep and narrow rural roads. With 217 ultra nuts, there were plenty of happy faces to have the chats with. The topic of training came up. The handful around me couldn't believe I did all my training independently, without a training group, or at least a training partner to meet with and ensure my attendance. I agreed, having someone expecting you to show up is a positive influence, pushing you to make it when you don't feel like it, but I liked the freedom of being my own boss. I had a demanding schedule, and it was hard enough to fit my running around my own commitments, never mind having to try to work it around other people's commitments too. I could stick my runners on whenever I wanted and run at my own pace. Some days I ran in silence, listening to the nature of the Phoenix Park and the rhythm of my breathing and footsteps; if I wanted some distraction from my thoughts, I'd stick on the radio and plug in the headphones. I'd be the only runner on the challenge itself, so it suited me down to the ground and made sense to train solo to get used to my own company.

The 64-kilometre run went smoothly, bar the ending when I got a bit excited, and let loose a little when we returned to some civilisation. It wasn't like the Dublin Marathon, with crowds pretty even throughout. Connemara is remote. All the spectators were concentrated near the finish, as the ultra participants started merging with the half and full-marathon participants. Once I started seeing people on the roadside, I could feel myself speed up a little. I felt like I was moving at a similar pace to the five-kilometre beach run, at the end of the sprint triathlon, enjoying the process of passing some people out. Most participants were struggling and slowing at the end, where I felt like I had loads left in the tank, having run a reserved pace throughout. I had forgotten Gerry's wisdom not to take my eyes off the ball. The goal was to complete 35 marathons in 35 days. It wasn't about running consistent sub-four-hour marathons or doing one three-hour marathon in the middle of the 35. It certainly wasn't about trying to run a fast last five kilometres of a training ultra.

I paid no attention to my watch or pace while running, just doing what felt comfy. Still, it was reassuring to see steady splits at the end – my first half-marathon split in 2 hours and 19 minutes, second half-marathon split in 2 hours and 23 minutes and third half-marathon split in 2 hours and 28 minutes, for a total time of 7 hours and 11 minutes. Pretty damn terrifying hearing of the Italian winner, Giorgio Calcaterra, finishing in under four hours!

With 5,208 calories burned, according to my GPS watch, I leapt on my Dad, who was patiently waiting, laughing with joy to see me sprint across the line with a smile. The proof was in the pudding, and we now knew I was ready to rock 'n' roll for the 35-marathon challenge, although there was an unfamiliar issue with the sole of my foot which seeded some doubt. Never mind, for now, it was time to enjoy a humongous pizza and beer with Dad.

BOY'S TRIP

With the bulk of my training complete, weekly kilometre totals were on a downwards trajectory but still required over 160 kilometres per week during the next three-week block. First though was a much-needed recovery week, with 'only' 95-kilometres to be completed. I was moving gingerly on my foot once the effects of the Connemarathon kicked in. I decided it best to run even less than what was programmed. I was too close to the start line to push through this kind of pain and risk the entire challenge.

With time freed up somewhat, it didn't mean resting on

my arse or heading to the pub. To make the most of the injury break, my father insisted we check out the route. He thought I'd be stupid to head off relying solely on the support crew, not knowing where I was going myself. Initially, I was reluctant. A fun part of the challenge was the unknown and seeing new places on foot. I had been fortunate enough to be taken by my parents to the Eifel Tower in Paris and the Colosseum in Rome, but there were swathes of Ireland I hadn't yet seen. I'd never set eyes on the Giant's Causeway, Newgrange or the Cliffs of Moher. Driving the route first, took away the romantic notion of exploring and discovering as I ran.

Not being able to do much running with my foot in bits, I trusted in Dad's wisdom, and off we headed in his car. Starting back in Waterford, we went over to Wexford and all the way up the east coast to Ballycastle on the north coast. We were stopping every 42.2 kilometres, cross-referencing each point with my map and distance markers. We wanted to be confident in the route and the daily marathon distances. It was one thing to have the distances add up on my Google Maps printouts and Map My Run, but it was no harm triple checking on the ground against the car's odometer. I didn't want to do 34 marathons and find myself still halfway up the country, instead of being on the start line for the Waterford Viking Marathon finale. Whenever we came to crossroads that might cause confusion, I made sure to pay attention and took notes to minimise the risk of future errors.

After three days on the road, we had to get back. The first 25 days were scoped out, and the distances on the ground matched the paper maps I had printed out for each day. Not having time to check the last 10 days meant I would still see something new, down around Kerry and through Cork, which gave me a reward to work towards. My dad knew Ireland's roads and towns like the back of his hand, having attended countless football and hurling matches through the years. Driving these distances was nothing to him but I was stiff as a board from sitting in the passenger seat. *Christ, what's it going to feel like to bloody run all that?* It was a helpful exercise to appreciate the actual distance I would have to journey on foot.

Having come so close to losing Dad to the stroke, I was still hyperconscious that our time together could be our last and made sure I cherished our boy's road trip. I'd taken for granted a lot of time with him before the stroke because it didn't feel finite. *Sure, I'll see him next weekend, won't I?* That attitude was gone. We smiled, chatted, listened to his Sharon Shannon CDs, taking in Ireland's rural and coastal sights, present and enjoying each other's company.

IF IT 'AINT BROKE, DON'T FIX IT

Trying to resolve my Connemarathon foot injury, I went to Siobhan for physio treatment and even got an MRI. To my relief, nothing major showed up on the scan and rest was recommended. Despite the injury, I was keen not to lose the fitness I had worked so hard to accumulate. I just had to work around the pain and keep ticking over on the stationary gym bike and rower, mixing in some weights, mobility, and flexibility. It was a bit dull and frustrating compared to the trails, but it was a necessary evil to keep the show on the road.

I thought the recent change in the brand of runners was too coincidental. I compared them to the Nike Pegasus I had worn up until April. The new runners' soles were much narrower in the middle, where the arch of my foot would rest. The arch was where the pain was affecting me the most. As my dad would say, 'if it ain't fixed, don't broke it!' It was a rookie mistake, wearing fresh runners for the ultramarathon without a few trial runs to break them in. More generally, there was no point changing footwear that I knew worked for my feet, if I was able to avoid it, especially so close to the event itself. I contacted my clothing sponsor, but they didn't sell Nike runners, so I got in touch with Alfie Hale Sports; my local sports shop that I had been going to since I was a child. Thankfully, they were more than willing to help me, and we made a trade. I did a straight swap of all my new shiny runners for cheaper pairs of Nikes. Another problem resolved. I just had to show patience with my damaged body, before starting to get back running and breaking each new pair of runners in on rotation.

CATWALK

The fundraising efforts that were above and beyond the call of duty were continuing full steam ahead. My childhood neighbour and friend Aisling Kennedy conceived the idea of a fashion show, putting on a great night, with local shops and friends all getting involved. Walking down a catwalk and doing a twirl was the last thing I expected to be doing when I signed up for the lap of Ireland run. Still, after my interactions with the charity, it seemed clear the run alone would not be enough to entice the public to donate their hard-earned cash. The show required massive effort – tickets, posters, event advertising, seating, balloons, lighting, sound system, DJ, volunteer participants, clothes, master of ceremonies. With my hotel workplace providing the venue at a favourable rate, the evening was a success and another €1,000 was added to the kitty. All these components of media work and spin-off fundraisers, like football tournaments, a fashion show, a comedy night, cake sale, raffles and pub quizzes, required lots of time I hadn't anticipated. They were energy-draining distractions from training and college, but were necessary to achieve a respectable fundraising total in the absence of any corporate donations. *No corporate donors: the event is doomed,* was the message I got from the charity. *That is that so,* seemed to be their defeatist attitude. Leaving this as a conclusion didn't sit well with me, and the only solution seemed to be doubling down on the grassroots fundraising drive. At least playing a role in organising the local initiatives felt like I was trying my best, instead of prematurely flailing my hands in the air in defeat because fundraising was more challenging than expected.

With four weeks to the start of the run, my final-year college dissertation was coming due and exams were nearing. It was stressful. I took great comfort, though, in the body of training I had accomplished throughout the year. Since October, I'd amassed 10 marathons, including some ultramarathons over 48 kilometres, as well as completing consistent shorter runs in between these notable peaks. Although there were moments that I was beaten and bruised, I survived it and was stronger for it. I earned the sureness that I'd make it to the start line, ready to attack the next phase of the journey, the actual 35-marathon challenge itself, or so I thought, the excitement making me forget the other variables.

UP SHIT CREEK

I felt hopeful in April, seeing the news of two lads raising over €16,000 for Special Olympics Ireland, running five marathons in five consecutive days, from Limerick to Dublin – 'Challenge 126' was the name they gave to the initiative, based on the distance being 126 miles. That had been the previous year. This year, I saw they were back doing the same route, but covering it over 40 straight hours instead of five days. This raised over €25,000. *That's very promising given the scale of my run in comparison*, I thought. *I should be able to get to €35,000 doing 35 marathons.*

However, there was another blow to challenge my optimistic outlook. Thankfully, I was used to jumping hurdles all my life and had worked too hard to build up steam on this train.

Dad pulled through, delivering on the charity's request from September. He got the formal permission for the Heart Foundation to do their bucket collection in the Aviva Stadium. The run was scheduled to start on the 27th May 2012 and the bucket collection was planned for the night before. It would be the last home game before the Boys in Green, and their Green Army would be on the march to Poland for the Euros. The friendly was bound to be a sell-out and should raise a rake of money for the charities. The permission was great news and another reminder of how lucky I was to have Dad back close to his former self, pulling out all the stops to help us run a successful project.

I was proud of him. He was helping me, of course, but he

was an unofficial ambassador for stroke survivors as well. Dad was personifying what was possible with a F.A.S.T. stroke response and a robust rehabilitation programme, using his gift of time to enable money and awareness to be given back to stroke charities. It was clear his contribution and involvement were making him feel good, which transferred to me – a feel-good purpose for us both.

Fulfilling our commitment to getting the stadium permission, I passed the fantastic news to the Irish Heart Foundation to work their magic. They were delighted, until we were just days out and they told me they'd secured only one volunteer bucket collector. There would be 52,000 delighted football fans in the stadium, and this was all they could muster to capitalise. It was demoralising.

The fundraising professional told me I should get friends and family to step up and volunteer. *No shit! Because the charity has one person secured in the last eight months!* I thought. At this stage, I felt like telling them to get stuffed if they were willing to completely snub an opportunity like this and leave us high and dry at the last minute. Worse, this was their brainchild, but when they got the FAI's permission to collect at a sold-out match, they weren't prepared.

My dissertation was now due and exams were kicking off. I had enough stress to deal with, without this shitstorm. I couldn't understand why they were reneging on what they signed up for. It felt as though they didn't want the money. How else could I explain a no show, when previous charities managed to raise thousands from well-orchestrated collections there? Not even any of the staff would step up. It fell outside their nine-to-five work responsibilities. My efforts felt ever more underappreciated as I was left to salvage this event to benefit their cause. *Again, why am I running thousands of kilometres to chip in towards their salary, and fixing this botched collection for them, if they won't bother shaking a feckin' bucket themselves or even find other volunteers?*

They'd clocked me firmly on the chin. I was on wobbly feet but not knocked out. I could not control the overpromising and underdelivering of another person. It didn't seem fair or right. No amount of fighting back or complaining would change their actions or conclusions. That would just be wasted energy on my part. It was what it was, and I needed to get on with it, without relying on their help. I had the option to see a great opportunity wasted – or to do something constructive about it. I felt that my dad and I had been disrespected and left looking bad. I didn't want to pass the same show of disrespect onto the FAI, who had generously facilitated the charity's request. It would seem like we lacked integrity if we walked away so late. I couldn't imagine associating myself with one lousy volunteer in a 52,000-person stadium. That would be shameful.

Studying was put on ice and I went to glue the pieces together, calling friends and family, with steam blowing out of my ears. I just wanted to be bloody running and not dealing with this crap anymore.

My receding hopes that the charity would sort the logistics in time were dashed when the clock had reached a deadline. I would have had zero physios along the route if it weren't for Siobhan's 'can-do, will-do' attitude getting several of them in place. The charity had no meal arrangements and little over a handful of nights' accommodation. Oddly, despite the fact that they had known we were a three-person running team for eight months, they only booked us rooms with two single beds, leaving one of us to sleep on the floor during the sparse number of nights they had arranged a roof over us. What a shambles!

Because of all the undelivered components from the logistics standpoint, the senior fundraising professional from the Heart Foundation proposed that I defer my 35 marathons until the following summer. That way, they could be a bit more organised on logistics and fundraising. Amid my final weeks of college and the looming start of the challenge, I couldn't believe the words I heard over the phone. My stomach bubbled to a sickening boil as my temperature rose with blood flushing to my cheeks, fighting the urge to hang up the phone. I'd just about had enough. *Next year? Next year!? Are you fuckin' kidding me!?* is what I screamed in my mind. You just couldn't make it up! As if I had nothing better to do than repeat the thousands of anti-social kilometres on my own so I could give him a second chance at keeping his word!

With that proposition sinking like a lead balloon, he didn't give up but changed the angle of attack. To try to entice me to defer and buy them more time to take another stab at it, the fundraiser even suggested I change the challenge to running eight marathons in eight European countries over the course of the following year instead. He thought the prospect of travel abroad might sway things.

'Never work with animals or children,' is the saying. At

that point, I felt like you could quite easily add charities to the list. *Cowboys, Ted*. It showed how little the individual valued the effort I had put in throughout the year, painstakingly preparing my body and mind to run 35 marathons in 35 consecutive days, starting the 27th May 2012. They failed to grasp how much running a lap of Ireland meant to me and the urgency I felt to complete the challenge as soon as possible.

I was primed to be let loose on the roads, and my dad had fought his way back to life. Without a split second of thought, I told him there wasn't a hope in hell I was cancelling or deferring my marathon challenge. I'd fulfilled my end of the bargain. He hadn't. That was on him, not me. His word meant nothing at that point anyway. I wasn't going to risk another year of my life in their hands, which on the face of it would likely end in a similar conversation one year later. I had no evidence to believe otherwise. I told him I'd sort the logistics myself with the handful of days I had left. *I'll find a way under, over, through or around.* There was no lack of will on my part, so I'd bulldoze a path if I had to. *Fuck 'em, so,* was my combative attitude at that point. *I'll show them how to get a job done.*

Once I knew it was all on me and in my control, it was actually a relief. No more thinking, *I wonder if they sorted this or sorted that?* As undesirable and concerning as the task at hand was, I knew I'd pull it out of the bag. I *had* to, but I only had a matter of days to try to patch the leaks the charity hadn't been able to plug over eight months.

The charity had estimated the expenses would exceed €15,000 and they hadn't found an overarching cash sponsor or a group of smaller sponsors, since September. I was a full-time student doing a menial, part-time, minimum-wage job. I couldn't self-finance the adventure. Having a student bank account meant I didn't even have the option to irresponsibly pay for it with debt, as I wouldn't qualify for a loan or credit card. I was up shit creek without a paddle, but retreating was not an option.

These are the project-management stresses people don't necessarily think of when they hear of a person running a lap of Ireland. I was in the same boat initially, thinking, *all I need is the training plan. It'll be grand.* The charity took planning, organising and funding responsibilities from me, with the view that this challenge was marketable and Irish businesses would leap at the opportunity. We thought, with corporates covering the expenses, I'd just need to run 1,500 kilometres to generate online donations from the public. Simple on paper. It was naive of the experienced fundraising professional and me, although I felt I at least had a reasonable excuse. I thought they should be much better positioned to forecast this eventuality and flag unrealistic expectations from the outset. At least then, we could have prepared for the possibility of no corporate funding. I was on a steep learning curve about the joys of the real world.

With the mountain of logistics before me, I would do everything in my power not to fall at the last hurdle. Running had to take a back seat as the challenge quickly approached. Rather than a measured training taper period, I was effectively running shag-all. I had to accept that it didn't matter if I was in the shape of my life and able to run forever. Unless the logistics support was in place, I couldn't even start. I had to sacrifice my fitness and physical preparedness – and risk my degree – to get the house in order.

The Heart Foundation had done a fantastic job on the website, with my childhood friend Darren Doheny providing slick photographs that made me look like I knew what I was doing. Dad's work to arrange the photocall with Giovanni Trapattoni created some media profile and added credibility, with the charity's Communication Manager spreading it far and wide, coordinating great coverage. I had to hope that was enough to get some buy-in from business, with time rapidly running out to get organised.

Although I managed to source a support car with plenty of time, the charity couldn't find anybody to do the vehicle branding. I explained the situation to my flatmate, Simon, a graphic design student. He immediately created the Heart Foundation lettering and logo to stick on the car, along with the website donation link. Just days later, we stood proudly, admiring the work – a slick branded car parked in the driveway of my family's home. Despite the mess under the event's bonnet, at face value we appeared to be a serious operation now.

My father got in touch with the owners of the Horse and Hound Hotel, who he knew from his days working with Heineken. I was due to finish day one's marathon right on their doorstep in Ballinaboola, County Wexford. They were more than happy to help the sporting endeavour, their daughter Gráinne Murphy being a 2012 Olympic swimmer. Providing food and accommodation was not a problem for them either.

Except for the full schedule of team members and the

car, my Excel spreadsheet was mostly blank. Like staring at my initially daunting training plans, I needed to remain composed. There were many hotels, meals and physios yet to sort but a box at a time would see the problem steadily resolved. Cutting it fine, I managed at least to get day one's boxes filled – two team members, a branded support car, food and accommodation for three. That meant I could get the show on the road anyway. With some space to sigh relief, I took a retreat to the local countryside for a short five-kilometre run, to cram, and to reward myself with some calm and silence.

It was the day of the sell-out pre-Euros match and the farcical stadium collection – one day before the run started. With the handful of days I was given to salvage things, I mustered together 12 friends to add to the charity's one volunteer. The lads were troopers, coming in at the last minute and giving up their time, but with tens of thousands of fans in attendance, they just didn't have the numbers to do the opportunity justice and were only able to cover one small section. Unlike preceding charity collections in the Aviva, we fell way short of their €8,000 hauls and came in with a meagre €900. It was a kick in the balls, but I knew I had done the best I could in the dire situation and knew my friends had given their all too.

Although I had only been planning to give the NRH and Football Village of Hope a 20% share, I now felt it was unfair to those causes. They were only getting 10% each – of €900 – from the stadium collection. They should have been getting 10% each of €5,000 plus. I had had enough of being let down. I reduced the Heart Foundation's stake from 80% of the pot to 66% and decided to split the remaining portion evenly between the other two charities. I wanted to keep my word to them about getting the majority share, but I couldn't reward their careless attitude to wasting such a valuable opportunity.

I was fed up with the charity aspect, exhausted and dejected, wanting to simply run. Thankfully, I had made it through the year's training just about in one piece, scrambled the start of the event together at the last minute and, ready or not, I was about to lace up to try to become what I wanted to be.

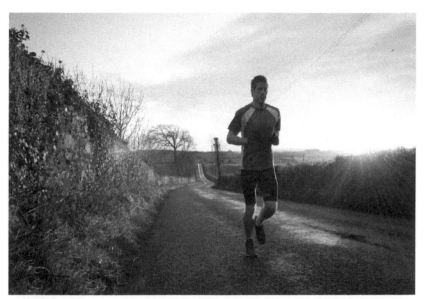

Clocking up the training miles on the back roads from Waterford City to Tramore.

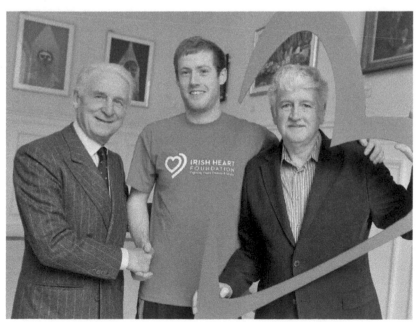

The 35-marathon press launch with Dad and the former Republic of Ireland football team manager, Giovanni Trapattoni.

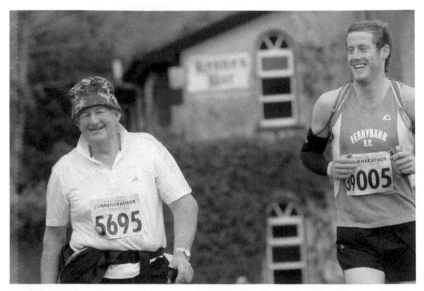

Enjoying the 64-kilometre Connemarathon ultramarathon training session, April 2012.

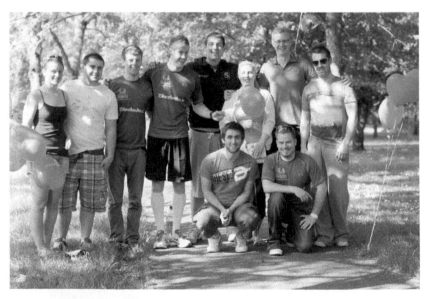

Marathon 1: With friends at the start line in the People's Park, Waterford City. Back row, from left to right: Grace Doyle, Niall Moran, Seán Drohan, me, Stephen O'Rourke, Aisling Kennedy, Simon Cody, Eddy Killeen. Front row, from left to right: Darren Doheny and Tom Davies.

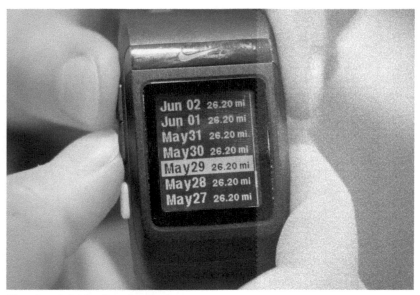

Marathon 7: 26.2 miles, day in, day out.

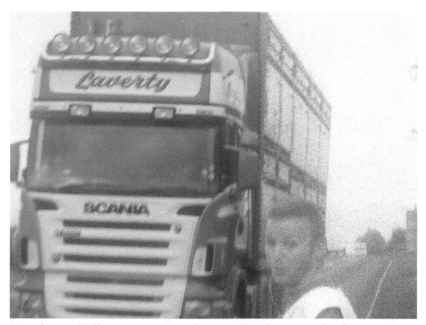

Marathon 11 (Ballymena to Ballycastle): Sean Kinsella running his first marathon on 'the most dangerous marathon' route.

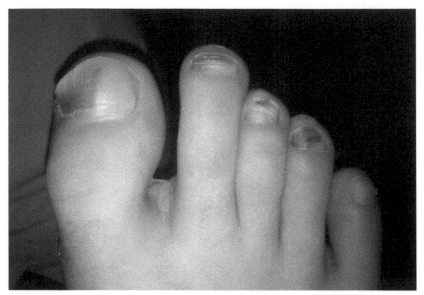

Marathon 14: Blisters and bruising.

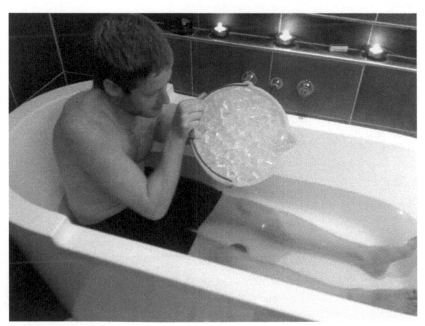

Marathon 18 (Ballina): Candlelit ice bath at The Ice House Hotel.

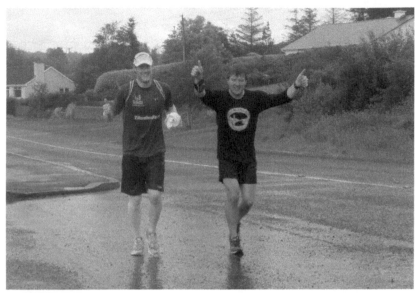

Marathon 19: Running in the rain with Alan Murphy.

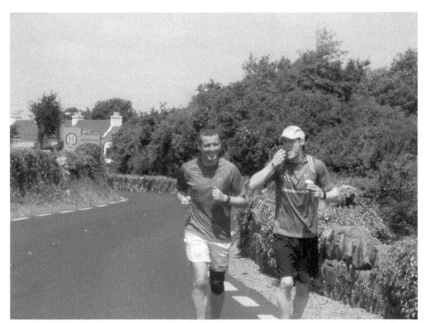

Marathon 22: Gorging on ice-cream with Ev, while passing through Ballyvaughan.

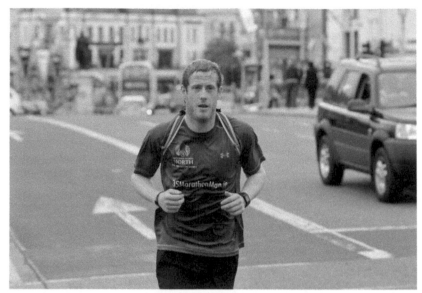

Marathon 31: Saint Patrick's Street, Cork City.

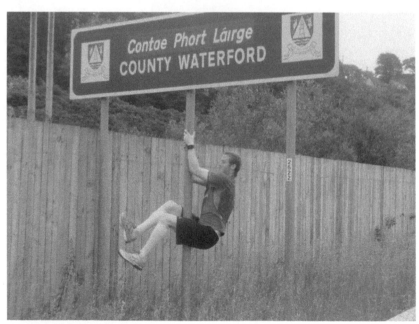

Marathon 32: A bit happy about reaching County Waterford.

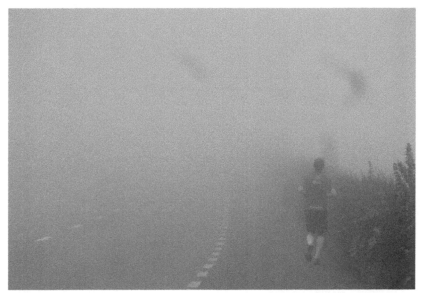

Marathon 32: Running into the fog and hoping cars don't use the hard shoulder.

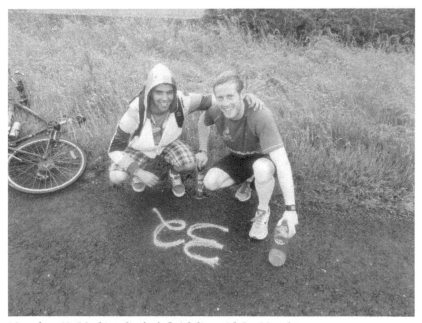

Marathon 32: Marking the day's finish line with Joe Murphy.

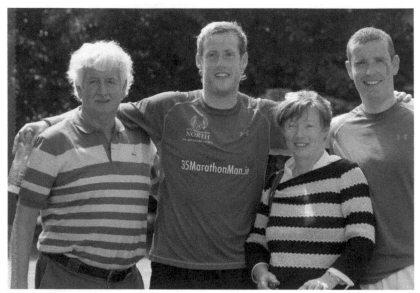

Marathon 34: Completing the lap of Ireland with my family supporting me.

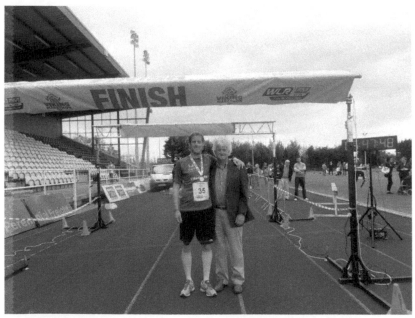

Marathon 35: The finish line of the Waterford Viking Marathon with Dad.

SIX
READY TO ROCK

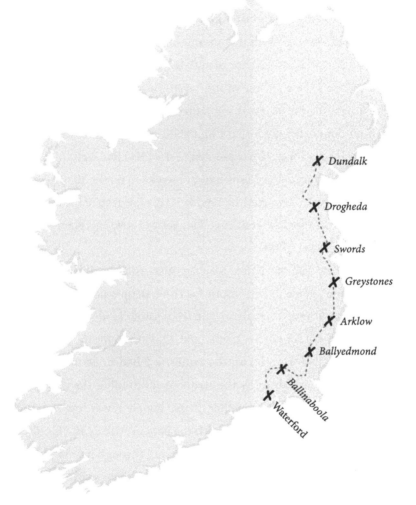

DAY 1 - DAY 7:

Waterford–Ballinaboola–Ballyedmond–Arklow–
Greystones–Swords–Drogheda–Dundalk

MARATHON 1: 27ᵀᴴ MAY 2012

It's mad. I made it. I am actually feckin' doing this. Oh boy! It was so satisfying yet surreal. The journey to the start line was hard-fought-for – my life's most significant challenge since the point of my dad's stroke. With the mountain of work completed, there was an overwhelming sense of satisfaction when the day finally came. It was the start line of the 1,500-kilometre run, but it was the finish line of the 3,000-kilometre couch potato to well-oiled runner boot camp. I felt that I had about 70 per cent of the work done and only about 30 per cent left to do. I had had eight months to do the 70 per cent and only had five weeks to do the 30 per cent, but that wasn't the point. I had made it this far despite the odds. I was buzzing. Plus, the challenge had yet to start, and people had already donated €4,000.

Come the start day, we had just under a third of the hotel rooms booked, with room for three people now. We had a beautifully branded Nissan on loan from John Flood's Dungarvan dealership and six physios confirmed. Only food for the first day, but hey-ho. Never mind all the running I had done up to that point, I was knackered by the stress of scrambling the stadium collection and logistics together. It was hugely rewarding to pull it off, keeping the dream alive with the help of friends and family. If it hadn't been for the adrenaline coursing through my veins, I'd have keeled over. In the previous few weeks I'd had a dissertation submission, exams, training, injury management and frantic project management. There was no time to rest or celebrate, with the long road ahead of me.

Everyone, me included, had underestimated the work in

getting to the start line. That was where the real challenge was for this test of endurance. Could I put the work in when nobody was watching and could I hold myself accountable day in day out? I'd stubborned my way to the start line – and I'd stubborn my way to the finish line.

Kick-off on day one was 10:30 a.m., dictated by the media call organised by the charity. It was later than I wanted, but after day one it would be up to me to decide my work schedule. When the launch day was out of the way, the plan was to start each day's marathon at about 08:30 a.m. The earlier start time would give me enough hours of daylight if things went pear-shaped but, more importantly, it would give my body time to heal. There'd be time in the day for normal mealtimes, liquids, ice baths, physiotherapy, stretching and a full night's kip. Starting late might risk running into the night, missing physio or dinner and messing up my typical sleep pattern. It was just easier to get up and get going without any dilly-dallying. I was drilled well in training so I wanted to keep the habit up.

I struggled through my porridge, force-feeding myself. It was a big day, and I hadn't an appetite, which was unusual for me. Tom Davies and Seán Drohan arrived in the support car, the vehicle loaded to the brim with our gear. There were heaps of runners that I would be wearing in rotation. I'd colour coded the laces so I could distinguish the otherwise matching white Nike Pegasus trainers. The plan was to wear the blue laces on day one, red laces day two, orange laces day three and white laces day four, then back to blue and so on. This was a tip from Gerry Duffy, to keep the runners functioning and avoid running one pair into the ground before starting to wear in the next. It seemed logical, so I went with it.

As well as runners, I had my compression socks, rising to just below my knees. The theory is that these improve blood flow, reduce muscle soreness and improve recovery. There were boxes of Jaffa Cakes, varieties of energy gels, Clif Bloks and Kellogg's Nutri-Grain Breakfast Bakes, bananas and crates of Lucozade Sport, ready to be diluted down with gallons of water that we had aboard too.

The sun was splitting the rocks, the windows were down and we chose to blare Bob Marley on our way to the start line. It was a carnival atmosphere that felt more like an ending than a start. I was happy out en route to the city's park, where the next leg of the journey was about to begin.

I got a great show of support from people coming down to wish me the best with my escapade. Mam, Dad, Ev, relatives and friends in a sunny park on a beautiful morning. What more could I want?

Once the photographers were finished, it was somewhat anticlimactic. *Right, I suppose I better get going so.* With a few more hugs and kisses, I slowly wandered out the park gates and made my way towards the bridge that leads out of Waterford. A random man was running beside me amongst a group of my friends. I briefly struck up a conversation with him as I didn't recognise him, and he hadn't introduced himself.

'I'm just here to see what pace you'll be running. That's fine. All the best now.' He abruptly stopped running and gave a wave after only jogging by my side for about 100 metres.

'He approved of the pace,' I laughed to the remaining group with a shrug.

I was joined by my friends and former sprint training partners Billy Ryan and Stephen Murphy, who saw me to the edge of the city. Stephen Hall, who had arranged the trade of sponsored runners, joined along for about 16 kilometres. Last but not least, was one of my former athletics clubmates and teammates from Tramore AFC, Alex Flynn, along for the full day's ride. He was an out and out distance runner and, although we had played football together loads, our paths had never crossed on the track. He had never done the marathon distance before. I was delighted my event made him decide it was time to tick it off his bucket list. He found the slowness odd. As a competitive distance runner, he was used to fast miles and the racing mindset. For me, the emphasis was moving forward while preserving my body as best I could for tomorrow's marathon. He'd run long distances but never spent this much time on his feet before. Luckily for me, I'd mastered the long slow run, so it was merely another day in the office. I had the knowledge that I could run 42.2 kilometres one day and 42.2 kilometres the next since I'd done it in training. Day one and day two were certain and to be enjoyed. It was days 3 to 35 that were the big question marks in my head.

I had a 10-minute break at the midway point, around New Ross, to do a radio interview trying to rally donations, but I didn't want them to become a standard feature. It dragged the run out longer than I wanted and disrupted the momentum but it did help the tally of funds donated online.

Tom and Seán were thrown in at the deep end as the

support crew. There was no formal induction or team briefing. We were long-time friends, happy to muddle through and to learn on the job. They'd spin a few kilometres ahead and pull in. We'd have a quick chat, or I'd grab some food or ask them to refill my hydration pack as I jogged on. Although I had the team there with drinks on hand, I was used to training with the hydration pack and preferred sipping away at the plastic tube when I needed it, rather than relying on and waiting to reach the team. The first day was bloody boiling for a pasty Irishman, which equates to 25–30°C for the rest of the world. I was burning through liquids like never before, since I knew I had bottomless refills. I went with a 50% water and 50% sports drink mix. The sports drink on its own was too concentrated and sweet, making me feel ill, but I had found the watered-down version suited me perfectly in training. On a shoestring, this also meant the expensive sports drinks lasted twice as long too.

There were some steady inclines on the first day, mainly out of New Ross. The temperature added a layer of difficulty, but it was pretty smooth sailing, if slower than anticipated, finishing in 4 hours and 51 minutes. Unlike my clockwork 4 hours and 30-minute training marathons, radio interviews and team check-ins delayed things a little. I didn't get too hung up on time. The main thing was I made it to the start despite the obstacles, had made it through day one and was near Ballinaboola, County Wexford, still feeling fit and healthy.

MARATHON 2: 28ᵀᴴ MAY 2012

Day two was a stark contrast to the previous day's atmosphere of family, friends and runners for company. It was just me, Seán, Tom and the open road. We returned to day one's finish line and were ready to roll a little before 08:30 a.m.

I took a wilderness pee on the roadside, embracing the freedom of adventure and unceremoniously started jogging along the car-dominated N25. We set our aim towards Wexford Town to the east, before we were due to make a turn and start our journey north.

The first half of the marathon felt comfortable and time flew as I ran through Wexford Town. Some fatigue started to set in around the 29-kilometre mark, but nothing I hadn't experienced a million times in training. After my untrained experience running the Dublin Marathon a few months back and difficulties overcome during the steep training block, the bar for feeling beat up was set pretty high. I felt a blister start to form on my right foot, at the base of my second toe. *You gotta be kidding me!* I'd run a gazillion kilometres in training over the past few months, notching up a heap of marathons and ultramarathons and never once did I experience a blister, despite all the puddles and rain I'd endured. There wasn't a drop of rain on day two, and my runners were well broken in. To make things more frustrating, I was wearing socks which I specifically bought because of their marketing; '1,000 Mile' socks that promised no blisters for 1,000 miles if you wear these. *Funny you should say that*, blistering on mile 45 of a 1,000-mile run. When given the option to laugh or cry, I had to laugh – *damn advertisers*. Let that be a lesson that paper doesn't refuse ink, and you shouldn't believe everything you read. I should have stuck with the worn-in training socks I was used to.

My namesake, Alan Corcoran from South East Radio, interviewed me while I kept on the go, not wanting to waste time loitering on the roadside like yesterday. The attempt at multitasking failed, and I had to stop so we could hear each other. Having halted the run, I found it problematic to get going again. The blister had become much more apparent when I started back running after the pause. I selected Roger Alan Wade's song on my iPod and began to sing in my best Tennessee accent as I got on with it.

'If you're gonna be dumb, you gotta be tough,

When you get knocked down, you gotta get back up.'

It was much to the amusement of the lads in the support car, who voiced some concern about me losing the plot so early in the challenge. This challenge was no walk in the park. I was hurting but knew maintaining a positive attitude would be in my interest and the teams.

Instead of driving a few kilometres ahead, stopping and waiting for me to catch up, they decided to stick near me for the last five kilometres for company. It made a big difference and added some fun to the mission, as they honked the horn, blasted nineties dance songs and threw a few awful shapes to make me laugh. With the branded car next to me, drivers surmised I wasn't just out for your typical jog and joined in with some beeps of encouragement too. Either that or they wanted us to get off the road and stop slowing up traffic!

I completed day two's marathon in 5 hours and 10 minutes. All my training marathons had come in at 4 hours and 30 minutes and the fact I was off the comfortable training pace was bugging me. I certainly felt worse for wear after day one and day two compared to the faster back-to-back training marathons I did in March. *It's not about the times; it's about finishing*, I reminded myself, as I tried not to worry about the unexpected slowness. I hadn't been as consistent in my training during the weeks leading up to the challenge, with life and organisational responsibilities taking over. I convinced myself that my body just needed time to reawaken and readjust to the daily long runs.

MARATHON 3: 29TH MAY 2012

On day three, I began running in Ballyedmond, a few kilometres south of Gorey. The 8:30 a.m. start worked perfectly, and I decided I'd keep the routine going. It allowed plenty of time for the essentials. My routine would generally look like this:

7:00 a.m.

Get up, start drinking my litre bottle of water, stretch and pack up my bags.

7:45 a.m.

Get funny looks off the accommodation staff for ordering two bowls of plain porridge for breakfast while watching the lads indulge in full fry ups. *Bastards!*

8:15 a.m.

Leave the hotel or guesthouse and drive to the point where I finished the previous day's marathon. Wait for my GPS watch to pick up the signal.

8:30 a.m.

Start the 42.2-kilometre run and try to finish without
injuring myself too severely, ideally in a time between
4 hours and 30 minutes and 5 hours and 30 minutes.

1:00 p.m.–2:00 p.m.

Finish the marathon, have a protein shake and a peanut
butter sandwich, then drive straight to the hotel for an ice
bath or jump in the sea (if it was nearby), followed by
a glorious warm shower.

3:00 p.m.–4:00 p.m.

Drive to whatever pub, hotel or restaurant was kind enough
to sponsor some grub for us and enjoy the company of my
friends. The vast majority of the team members were not
runners and had little or no interest in running, so once
I ran the marathon, it was nice to completely switch
off until the next one.

05:00 p.m.

Physio.

06:00 p.m.–07:00 p.m.

Drive to whatever pub, hotel or restaurant was kind
enough to supply dinner.

08:00 p.m.–10:00 p.m.

Snack, stretch, ice the worst aches and pains. Try to update the event's social media page so that family, friends and the general public could follow along on the journey, feel sorry for me and donate to the charities.

10:00 p.m.
Light's out and sleeping like a baby.

Despite the abnormality of the routine when I thought about it, I was surprised by how easily it became normalised – just another day at this unique office.

It didn't take me long to realise my romantic notions of running to a new town and spending the remainder of the day exploring its nooks and crannies was just a pipedream. The run-centric schedule didn't allow time for distractions but, with hours pounding the pavement, I made sure to take in my natural surroundings as best I could.

The days were long, not just for me, but for the team too. I'd managed to salvage the organisation side of things just enough to get the show on the road, but I hadn't secured food beyond day one and was short of 23 nights of accommodation that I couldn't afford to pay for. Tom and Seán were doing great work from the mobile operations centre. While I ran, they sorted logistics on the go, building off my route printouts and basic Excel spreadsheet with a handful of entries. Tom went about upgrading the spreadsheet immediately. Loves a good Excel that accountant!

With a polished spiel prepared, they went about calling hotels, B&Bs, bars, restaurants, cafés and physios in the locality of the finish, asking politely if they were willing to help out. Once the nearest day was locked in, they'd move to the next and the next. Like trying to find a job as an inexperienced graduate, it was a case of persistence but the team wasn't long getting most vacant slots filled in with the right tone and pitch. I could have kissed the pair of them. The lack of results throughout the year had been a real worry, especially since I had bulldozed ahead regardless. The lads were getting it done with a smile and while chucking Jelly Babies out the window at me. I was now in reliable hands and didn't have to be concerned about sleeping rough or surviving on protein shakes and cereal bars. Tom and Seán wouldn't let it come to that.

The beauty of the run was that each day we were 42.2 kilometres further up the road, usually in a different county and at least in another town or city. We weren't hitting up the same establishments twice. Most businesses were more than happy to give one night's accommodation or a meal for three to contribute to the effort, in return for a mention on the event's Facebook page. We'd be gone out of their hair the next day and hassling the next community for support. The quick success rate of Tom and Seán meant I had no excuses anymore. Logistics were firmly in hand. It was entirely up to me now to keep moving and look after my end of the business. Finally, I could just focus on running again.

There was poor visibility at the start of day three, car after car speeding along the narrow roads, causing me unease. When you think about road running, traffic danger doesn't spring to mind (unless you're my mam). Given the road layout, Irish weather and some people's driving style, a road collision was a real and serious threat. Luckily, this had crossed my mind at some point, and I'd packed a hi-vis vest for the journey. It wasn't the most stylish rigout but better safe than sorry!

There were some nipple issues eight kilometres in. I learned while training that chafing nipples were real and, feck me, can get very sore. Before day three of the challenge, it had only occurred on one long run in the depths of winter. It had been perishing out, the wind blowing a gale and the rain hitting me head-on – the triple threat of conditions for nipple chafe. When far from home in training, there was little I could do but endure the stinging sensation, damning the gods as the poor guys were chiselled away. My nipples were blessed on marathon three, though, with the privilege of a support team! Not wanting to end up with two bloodstreams down my blue event t-shirt, I asked the men to ready my tools, stat – razor, tub of Vaseline, sticky plasters.

'What are you going at?'

'They don't teach you this craic in college. Give me space to work.'

The guys were in stitches as passing traffic wolf-whistled me as I trimmed enough chest hair to ensure the band-aids would stick. I could well take the jeers. This challenge was already grim enough without adding raw nipples to the equation.

I had to start concentrating intently to hold form as I ran, trying my utmost to ignore the blister I instinctively wanted to keep the pressure off. With great distances, it's not the large rock you stump your foot on that will necessarily be your demise, but the tiny pebble that repeatedly wears on you. During training, I learned that if I tried to run pain-free by altering my technique to account for whatever it was that was hurting, it tended to throw something else way out of whack, multiplying my problems. As hard as I felt I was trying to ignore the blister's pain and plant my foot like usual, it mustn't have worked as the pain in the arch of my right foot was growing.

The Gorey natives beeped me on from their cars, the encouragement helping me tolerate the pain a bit better. I had to resort to walking more than I wanted to, especially over the last six hilly kilometres, after Arklow Town towards Brittas Bay. The walking felt like it was taking the strain off my banjaxed foot but prolonged the time I had to spend putting weight on it. It was a tricky balancing act.

Although hurting, I enjoyed the sense of achievement conquering the unknown, three marathons in three days. 'Only 32 to go lads, we'll be there in no time,' I joked with Tom and Seán. I completed marathon three in a personal record slow time of 5 hours and 20 minutes; the trajectory of my times was not looking too positive. Rather than worry or moan, I focused on the present and what I might be able to do to make things better. With the sea next to me, a refreshing dip was the best thing for the body and soul so in I hopped, with my recovery sandwich in my hand!

MARATHON 4: 30ᵀᴴ MAY 2012

While I lacked appetite on morning one, once the excitement and emotions dissipated, I was eating like a horse. I craved calories from the second I woke, making light work of my two bland porridge mountains each day before hitting the road. I then began grazing roughly every 30 minutes or so. It wasn't an exact science, just whatever I felt I needed: a banana, Jelly Babies, Jaffa Cakes, energy gels, cereal bars or Clif Bloks. In conjunction with the loose feeding strategy, I made sure to keep sipping the diluted energy drink from my hydration pack.

The team worked hard to secure local food sources as I ran. Beggars can't be choosers, so we took what was given, whether soup and sandwiches, a one or two-course meal, and more often than not, the whole nine yards, dessert included. Whatever we could get, we were extremely appreciative of the support. With my empty student pockets and no cash sponsors, the run would have been a disaster without the goodwill of Ireland's local businesses.

Day four began about a kilometre south of Brittas Bay and the route brought me through Wicklow Town, Kilcoole and Greystones. Before getting going, I made a dismal attempt at taping up my injured foot, trying to relieve the strain and keep the ever-slipping blister plaster in place. Despite my deteriorating condition, I was able to enjoy the pleasant countryside views along the back roads and settled at a pace that caused the least discomfort whilst keeping forward momentum.

Now, on top of food and accommodation planning, Seán wanted to leave the comfort of the car to stretch his legs and join in for a few kilometres to see what all this running craic was about. He was a welcome distraction from the growing aches and pains, with my attention turning to him instead of my ailments. We chatted and laughed our way along, the kilometres disappearing behind us with a bit more ease.

To Seán's credit and my surprise, he joined me from kilometre eight, all the way to kilometre 32. That's no joke for someone without any running background at all. It also indicated how slow I was moving, but any ego had to be kept at bay. Slow and steady was the name of this game.

Tom and I had a right laugh watching Seán once he stopped, hobbling and cursing while helping to get my bits and bobs ready at my refuelling stops as my marathon continued.

'I'm fucked. It's not funny, lads,' Seán laughed.

It was kind of funny, though. Seán certainly got a much better impression of what this whole thing entailed, better able to relate to my experience. I felt good being responsible for getting someone else moving a bit more, although I did feel somewhat guilty laughing at the suffering I'd inflicted too.

Tom wanted in on the action as well, having seen what Seán had achieved. I hadn't seen Tom exercise since our days of playing chase on the streets as kids, except for nightclub dancefloors – but that's not the most transferable of cross-training. He didn't last quite as long as Seán. After about three kilometres, his feet got sore, and he sensibly retreated to the support car, surviving to guide the team for the rest of the day.

I joke, but the guys impressed me by getting out of the car and giving it a go. I appreciated the effort and the company. Having the lads there, chatting away for all those kilometres made the day fun and tricked my brain into paying less heed to the suffering I was going through.

Seán's half-marathon, was Tom's few kilometres, was now my ultramarathon. Everyone has their starting point. Remember, I hadn't been able to walk after my first marathon a couple of months before this. If you feel inclined to take up running after reading this, bear our experiences in mind and take it handy to start. Jumping into marathons and half-marathons without structured preparation will detract from the pleasure and health benefits running can give. Self-inflicted damage will deter most from lacing up again. Keep in mind, consistency trumps intensity. Start with a sensible distance, within *your* comfort range, not anyone else's. As a rule of thumb, only increase the weekly distance by 10% (ish) if there's no adverse effect from the previous week. Make sure to dial it back every fourth week or so too, as nobody can indefinitely increase the workload each week without consequence. Better yet, join a local club or beginners' group for the social aspect and get experienced input from a qualified and experienced coach, so you're not left with guesswork.

My day's marathon concluded with a challenging hill climb out of Greystones. The final effort was made worthwhile to find my dad standing there with a smile and a sports drink to welcome me on arrival. Dad's surprise appearance hit me right in the feels, daily marathons heightening my emotions. My body was breaking down, and I was getting even slower, finishing marathon four in 5 hours and 38 minutes, but it was an enjoyable one, nonetheless, because of the company.

I had slept like a log after day one, day two and day three. I never remember sleeping so soundly. After day four, I awoke in the middle of the night, having not cut off my liquids early enough. As I tried to stand up from the bed, I was reminded of my body's inability to walk after October's Dublin Marathon, but this was worse. I likened the aftermath of that Dublin run to being tackled by Paul O'Connell. Well, this was like being run over by a bus. I felt like an arthritic 90-year-old, not a 21-year-old athlete. In the darkness, I inched towards the bathroom, fighting the urge to groan in agony and trying not to wake the guys. When I made it, I looked at myself in the mirror, hunched over, both hands on the sink for support.

'*Christ,*' I whispered, shaking my head and laughing.

I checked the time. It was 04:00 a.m. *Ugh, how am I going to be on the start line for another marathon in only four more hours!?* Having taken a leak, I grimaced as I shuffled back to bed, concerned. I made a mental note not to drink so close to bedtime to avoid such misery and doubt in the future. I hadn't the energy to worry any further about the state of play, as I conked out before my shattered head hit the pillow.

MARATHON 5: 31ST MAY 2012

The alarm sounded. *Ugh, ready or not, here I come.* I was still in bits, but there was a world of difference, having had a few more hours sleep. At least I could walk like a normal human, which hadn't been possible a few hours prior. I took a bit more time to stretch before breakfast, getting my body primed and the blood flowing.

Seán Drohan departed the team and my friend Sean Kinsella stepped in to fill the vacant position. It was a frustrating day from the start. My beautiful routine was ruined as it took my GPS watch an age to pick up the satellite signal. The watch was giving me real-time feedback of the distance I was covering and my speed. It was keeping a record of the routes covered and marathon times too. It was foolish not to have a plan B to measure and record the distance, but it was too late for that now. We just had to sit and wait, shoving my wrist to the sky as if it made a difference in searching for a signal.

It was wet and raining, which didn't help morale either. Although mostly recharged from yesterday's marathon, my body had been on a downward trajectory from day one, each day slightly more painful and slower than the last. The watch, the rain and the stiffness weren't helped by the fact that I was starting on a long incline, continuing my climb out of Greystones. My positive attitude was being tested already as I made the error of allowing myself to pay attention to the doom and gloom.

After five kilometres, I warmed up, and my movement became a lot less deliberate. I settled into my groove and began feeling hopeful again. Up until Dublin, there'd been little to no turns, and the route was simple and straightforward. We hadn't put any thought into the problems of negotiating a capital city with a support car until we got there. Hindsight's no sight. The situation was made worse by the silly timing for a crew change; poor Sean Kinsella was chucked in at the deep end as we all struggled to stay together and not get lost amidst the hustle and bustle of the city.

We took the first wrong turn in Killiney. I was frustrated with the lads for not guiding me right but bottled up the emotions instead of saying anything. We didn't loop back to correct ourselves as it would only put us out by a greater distance. Instead, we kept trucking forward, trying to figure another way north as we advanced.

By kilometre 13, I got to pass the National Rehabilitation

Hospital, but I couldn't enjoy the milestone as much as I wanted to, experiencing unfamiliar lower back pain. I'd never had any back problems before, and the unfamiliarity of it brought some anxiety. *What have I done to myself? What if this is the injury that derails me? Blisters on my toes? Fine. But I need my back!*

The arch of my right foot had been giving me issues since Wexford, but now my left foot was getting sharp shots of pain through it as well. Between my back and my beat down feet, I'd slowed to a walk.

Wanting to bandage myself together and take an anti-inflammatory, I looked for my team through the rain. The support car was nowhere to be seen amongst the city traffic, bus lanes and cycle lanes making it illegal for them to pull in. *I should have planned for this.* The rain poured, my iPod broke, and things were getting bleaker by the minute. By the time I found the lads, I had overshot another turn I was meant to take and was not in a good physical or mental state.

Once the anti-inflammatories kicked in, I was back in motion, running – at least until we hit Dublin City Centre. I lost count of the number of stops and starts for traffic and trying to figure out where to go. On the fly, we decided it best to get the bicycle off the back of the car for the first time and have Sean accompany me on it. Taking the car through our planned city centre route was near impossible with the one-way streets and limited space to pull in. I told Tom to go ahead, and I'd see him again on Summerhill, on the other side of the city, just off O'Connell Street.

It wasn't long until I had lost Sean somehow. In the

excitement, he'd kept cycling when I'd stopped at the red light. He was meant to be guiding me to run past the Irish Heart Foundation office, as they wanted a photo taken for media coverage since they didn't make the Sunday morning day one start. I was on my own and hadn't a clue how to get to their offices from where I was, but I roughly knew which way was north from the road signs. Being honest, I didn't care for a photo at that moment and didn't stress it. I thought, *If they wanted to be in a picture, they could have come to the start line on day one.* I had more pressing matters. My priority was keeping an eye out for Sean and trying to make it through the city to Tom without being hit by traffic.

I knew the broad direction of travel and followed signs to the centre. I found my way onto Nassau Street and had my bearings again but was concerned for Sean's whereabouts on the bicycle. Weaving in and out of jammed footpaths, I made my way up O'Connell Street where I saw Sean outside the General Post Office. Disaster averted.

'Well, fancy seeing you here, Al. You out for a run, ya are?'

We both just laughed at the predicament and kept trucking, linking back up with Tom to finish our eventful day in Swords.

I was steadily falling apart, slowing even further, completing the marathon in 6 hours and 4 minutes. Nonetheless, another one down. *Surely it can't get much sorer or slower,* I hoped. *When will I be over the hump, if there is such a thing?*

My toes, toenails and feet had taken a battering by the time I'd run to Dublin – five consecutive marathons. I hadn't had to endure these sensations in training, nor the swelling of my feet, which was a new symptom. Usually, I could slide into my runners without undoing my laces. When I took them off after my day's marathon and went to put them back on to enter a shop, my feet wouldn't fit. The idea of restricting my poor swollen feet to the confined runners was unbearable. I threw caution to the wind and ventured about barefoot instead. It was a stupid risk in hindsight and an eccentric look shopping for a laptop charger in the Jervis Centre, but it felt so much better – despite the glares of embarrassment from Tom and Sean.

'We're not with him.'

It wasn't long until security approached and asked me to leave the premises but not before we managed to pick up what we needed to keep the car-based office operational – all in a day's work.

MARATHON 6: 1ST JUNE 2012

Day six, I put my toe to the start line at the end of Sword's main street, aiming for just north of Drogheda. Given the steadily slowing times and increasing pain levels, I wasn't too enthusiastic for the hours ahead of me but kept an open mind.

Sean tagged along to run with me for a few kilometres as company, which was always welcome. I'd grown accustomed to training exclusively on my own but found the companionship made the time pass quicker and softened the perception of pain a little. My back was still giving me problems, along with the front of my right knee joining the party. I felt like a right auld crock with everything except my baby fingers feeling the effects of life on the road. Around kilometre 15 I put on a knee-support and took an anti-inflammatory while crossing my fingers. During this little break, I took the opportunity to replace my blister plasters which had slid off once again.

With Dublin City in the rear-view mirror, the shamrock green countryside started to re-emerge after Balbriggan and traffic eased off. My heart rate was lowering the further from the city I got and the deeper I travelled along the rural roads. I felt good coming into Drogheda, all things considered. I was ready to end the day without so much as a blip – but best-laid plans and all that. I lost Tom and Sean again, this time as I passed through Drogheda. Cities and towns were not our friends.

Having scoped out this part of the route with my dad, I remembered where to go, and I didn't waste time waiting for the lads to appear. I ploughed on, hoping they'd turn up. The GPS watch ticked to 42.2 kilometres and I found myself alone on the hard shoulder of the main road out of town, with the support car nowhere to be seen. *Ah, for feck sake lads!* I was tired and getting hangry. Luckily some construction workers were digging up the road not too far ahead. I asked them if I could borrow their phone for a second.

'Well, where the feck are ye?'

'You're alive, great! We lost you.'

'I know that. I'm finished. Can you come rescue me, please?'

'We lost you in town somewhere and panicked. Eh, Sean's after heading off on the bike to try find you. I'm in the car, but now I can't find him.'

'Some disaster. Have to get off this fella's phone. When you find him, head a few kilometres out of town on the main road. I'll keep an eye out.'

Next thing, my dad pulls in beside me.

'Great to see ya, Al.'

'You too. Wasn't expecting ya. Chatting to the guys?'

'Yeah, Tom told me where I might find you, and I left him to search for Sean. Could be worse.'

The lads eventually pulled up, apologising. It turned out they'd been watching some show on the laptop while waiting for me to tortoise alongside them but they missed me running past. I hadn't spotted them either, to be fair. When they felt I should have definitely passed by, they'd gotten worried and went searching separately – some eejits!

We survived to muddle our way through yet another day. Day six down, completed in 5 hours and 48 minutes. I was glad to be back on the right side of the six-hour mark, that was for sure.

MARATHON 7: 2ND JUNE 2012

The discomfort of the back and knee pain of days five and six had all but disappeared. My body seemed to be slowly adapting to the new routine. From when I finished my daily marathon, my mind was on recovering effectively. I adopted the RICE approach to recovering from injury – rest, ice, compression, elevation. I was chilling out after the marathons, with the weight off my feet as much as possible and making sure lights were out at least nine hours before my alarm was set to sound. 10-minute ice baths were part of the daily post-marathon ritual. In terms of compression, I ran with compression socks during the day and slept in compression leggings at night. I even wedged pillows under the end of my mattress to try to elevate my legs a fraction. On top of the RICE strategy, I had light physio most days and made sure to stretch myself and foam roll every single morning too. Then there was the food. I ate as much food as the day's local sponsors provided, with nothing capable of filling the bottomless pit. I wasn't sure if any or all of the measures worked, but I could see no harm in trying every recovery angle. Even if only one method saw a 0.5% improvement, it was worth making life a bit easier for the next day. Of all, sleep seemed to be the magic pill, and I was particular not to compromise it. No matter how damaged I was during the day, I was in disbelief at sleep's healing properties. I just stopped worrying about the marathon's injuries because I was waking up afresh every morning, with yesterday's pains being no prediction of today's aches. The exception to this was the blisters, which seemed like they would stay for the entire ride. With no days off, there didn't seem to be time for my sensitive skin to heal. As bad as the blisters were, they weren't going to kill me, and if they weren't going to kill me, I could keep moving forward. If all my efforts to heal myself failed, I had anti-inflammatory creams and a handful of anti-inflammatory tablets as an emergency stand-by if it was getting too much to handle.

The day's marathon started with the guys blaring Bill Withers, 'Use Me', out of the car window to wind me up. Wind me up, because it had become their repeat song of choice yesterday, and I made the mistake of asking them to change it after the fourth loud blast. They had probed, found a weakness, didn't forget and attacked my eardrums:

'You just keep on using me

Until you use me up

Until you use me up ...'

Nightmare. My torment made the lads happy as they screeched the words out the rolled down windows at 08:45 a.m.

'Use me! Yeah, Al! Use me!'

'Christ, I have a feeling this will be a long day.'

I'd endure this extra layer of suffering for them. I didn't have much choice as they crawled in first gear beside me. *Bastards.* As painful as the audio repetition was for me, I knew piss-taking and messing was the medicine to get through hardship for us all. It would have been a dull, dreary five weeks if everything was just blisters, joint pain and serious business.

I was joined today for the last 24 kilometres by David Costello, who I had met during the Connemarathon. As happy as I was to have him along for the ride, it was crap timing. I was warmed up and running comfortably until about kilometre 21 when my left quad began aching. *Typical.* Just as the knee and back corrected themselves, something else went. I hadn't had a niggle like this one before either. Because David had made the effort to come out and support me, I didn't want to slow my jog down or switch to a walk. I'm sure he wouldn't have cared if I needed it, but the least I could do is bloody run when a runner joined me. I said nothing and carried on as if all was fine, but the discomfort increased with each passing kilometre.

We finished off the day in Ravensdale, County Louth, along a countryside road, with trees and wildlife distracting me from the internal torment. With David there to spur me on, I'd shaved 20 minutes off yesterday's time, finishing in 5 hours and

25 minutes. My times were bounding back in the right direction, but I couldn't help but feel I should have eased off when my quad signalled amber.

To have a break from the boring ice baths, we took a spin to the picturesque Carlingford Lough and took a dip in the shade of the Cooley Mountains, next to the twelfth-century castle. As scenic as the lough, castle and surrounding fertile hills were, it wasn't the brightest of ideas, as I had to hobble across a lot of jagged rocks to get waist-deep, abusing my poor tortured feet even further. Would I ever learn to take the easier route?

Concerned for my leg, we went straight to the physio after the icy dip. After some poking and prodding, the physio – someone who'd done marathons and Ironman races himself – told me he'd typically recommend at least four days of total rest for an injury like this.

'You've strained your quad, and it will only get worse and worse the more repeat demands you put on it. Can you take any rest?'

'No can do: it's 35 marathons in 35 days. I'm only on day seven.'

With that, he gave me a light and relaxing massage. He didn't seem too hopeful for my prospects but wished me the best of luck for the days ahead regardless.

SEVEN

RUNNING THE NORTH

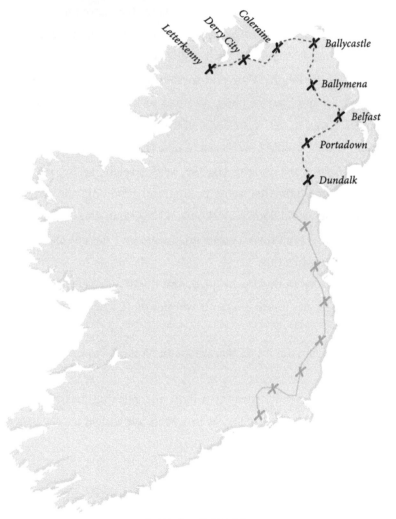

DAY 8 - DAY 14:
Dundalk–Portadown–Belfast–Ballymena–Ballycastle–
Coleraine–Derry City–Letterkenny

MARATHON 8: 3ᴿᴰ JUNE 2012

The Northern Ireland border was in sight. Well, the fireworks factory and a sign for currency exchange were in view. It was another little milestone. Without any thought, I'd set mini targets for myself. At the start, it was running more than three marathons back-to-back to achieve a new personal best; then it was geographical milestones like running to Dublin (marathon five), crossing to Northern Ireland (marathon eight) and so on. The short-term goal was to run today's marathon, which got broken down to running to the next tree if I was in a rough spot, physically or mentally. The ultimate goal was to make it to Waterford, but the gap between those was too much to contemplate, and I found these medium-range targets to be useful tools. There were no rewards, but there were milestones. I allowed myself a little pat on the back when I achieved them. I even told myself if I was really good and made it to Belfast, there'd be a nice cold pint waiting. Who needs a carrot on a stick when you have beer?

Day eight was a bit of a nightmare from the word go. My times were initially getting slower and slower with each passing marathon, but momentum had changed with two progressively faster marathons on day six and seven. I thought I was over the worst of the suffering and my body was adapting. I was hoping to get back to training's consistent time of 4 hours and 30 minutes. Wishful thinking! My body was in distress again today, particularly my feet and left quad. My right iliotibial (IT) band was flaring up too. The IT band is the connective tissue on the outside of the leg, between the knee and hip.

I tried to break up the run a little to seek bouts of relief. I started running for eight minutes and walking for two minutes. This was a strategy suggested to me by the physio in Dundalk. I didn't have the patience for it. I felt I'd be at this marathon all day if I kept that up. I spent the two minutes fixating on my watch and found it draining. I adjusted the strategy, taking a short walk after roughly every kilometre, without being controlled by the numbers on my wrist. I could forget about the run and the watch, taking in my surroundings instead. With a quick untimed recharge of my batteries, I'd get running again. I had to dig in but breaking it up into bite-sized pieces was the only way I was getting through this day. It was one of the most testing distance runs I'd ever done, and things certainly weren't getting any more comfortable as I had hoped for.

To make things even more interesting, we ran out of rural roads and were forced onto the motorway to continue north into Newry. Luckily it was a Sunday morning, so there was little to no traffic. Without much choice, the guys stuck on their hazard lights and veered into the hard shoulder, shielding me from any speeding northbound traffic. Having checked the maps, we knew it was only a short section. It was a matter of putting the head down to get out of harm's way as quickly as possible, hoping the police wouldn't stop us. It was definitively one of the most unnerving sections of the run up to this point. A motorway is not a sensible place for pedestrians.

We thought that was our fun done for the day until we got into Newry. Unexpectedly, we saw crowds of runners that looked to be part of a race. As we got closer, we discovered the Newry Marathon was on, and it was coinciding with my planned route.

The race meant Tom and Sean didn't have access to the roads for the support vehicle. Again, I was thankful Dad had insisted on us checking out the course in advance. I knew where I was and where I should be headed. Learning from our mistakes in Dublin, I grabbed my phone this time and waved goodbye to the guys, hoping to see them soon, as I improvised my way through the town, avoiding the masses of people.

As it was unexpected, we just made some quick spur-of-the-moment decisions to ensure my run continued. *The crowds seem to be in the start/finish area. Once I get around that little patch, we should be able to regroup on the other side of town.* When the support car wasn't appearing on the roadside, I gave them a call.

'What's the craic? I'm starting to get hungry and running a bit low on liquids here. Have you joined back up with the road yet?'

'We know where you roughly are, and we can see the route with the race runners on it, but we just can't get near it. The police stopped us and won't give us access. We've gotten as close to you as we're allowed, but we're probably a good eight kilometres ahead of you.'

We should have predicted this back in the town, but we had made our decisions in haste so as not to waste time and I hadn't taken food with me. Having slammed into the wall in training, I knew the sinking feelings and could sense my body slipping towards the hole. By chance, I found a chocolate Penguin bar from the previous night's B&B zipped in my back pocket. Those calories would buy me some time but not enough to reach the lads. With the roads closed and my team separated from me, I was left precariously in no-man's land with little option but to advance, my near-empty tank slowing my movements right down. Since the swarm of runners had already passed through this section of road, leaving a trail of waste behind them, I did what I had to do. Don't judge me! Ravenous and with nobody around, I spotted half a pack of Jelly Babies discarded on the overgrown grass verge, near some empty sports drink bottles and energy gel wrappers. It wasn't a high point in my life, eating someone's leftover floor jellies, but boy did they hit the spot. I was sweaty, sore and desperate, but the sugar stopped the tank from hitting empty and kept me moving in the direction of the roadblock, where the men would have some proper fuel for my depleted body.

Eventually, I spotted the lads, surrounded by the Police Service Northern Ireland. *What the feck have they done?* We're only in Northern Ireland a few hours. Apparently, the police were understandably dubious of the story Tom and Sean told them to try to gain entry onto the closed road. Feeding a Waterford man a banana didn't cut it as a plausible excuse in their books.

'Ah, would you look at that? You weren't codding us,' the police laughed as I staggered up to them.

I wasn't in any humour to engage with them, blaming the police for my deprived state. They fecked off after they got their laugh, and I could finally be like a kid in a candy store.

'I'll have one of everything, please, lads. One banana, one cereal bar, one caffeine tablet, one sports drink and a large Big Mac if you've got it?'

I know it sounds dramatic, but I had run over 330 kilometres in the past eight days, had missed two of the regular feeding points and had the added stress of not knowing exactly when I'd be reuniting with my team. It got relatively serious, relatively quickly.

My emotions were heightened, and I was ecstatic to see the guys and my food supply again. Replenished from gorging, we settled back to our routine without any police interference. The zapped energy and battle to safety had completely distracted me from any injuries. My mind had prioritised survival. With food and drink in me, my brain could focus once again on the pain. As predicted, my quad strain worsened, and my right shin and hay fever were pitching in now too.

Things improved for the last few kilometres, and they were enjoyable. This phenomenon seemed to be consistent, even back on the Tramore sprint triathlon, Dublin Marathon and Connemarathon. When the finish line came within reach, things became more manageable mentally and somehow that made things a bit easier on my body too. A big thing that lifted my mood was edging towards the physio massage and getting to eat desserts. Unlike the necessary hardship Rory put me through on the physio table earlier in the year, physio was always just a relaxing light touch during the challenge. There were no days of rest to heal up from any dry needling or deep tissue work, so it was just gently does it. After a long day on the feet, stressing the system, a nice massage was just what the doctor ordered, along with Death by Chocolate, ordered by me – whatever gets you through!

Unfortunately, on this occasion, we just had dessert scheduled but no physio. It was a Sunday, and I was getting further and further from home and any network contacts. I also learned there was some giant celebration for the Queen. Well for her, but this likely ruled out physio for the next day too. With this in mind and my body in a state of agony, I made sure to pay extra attention to my recovery, doing a little longer in the ice bath, a little bit more foam rolling, as painful as it was, and a bit more stretching.

Day eight was bleak, coming in with a hard-fought 5 hours and 56-minute marathon. Oddly, I was prouder of this run than I was any previous day. It was a real slugfest this one, the hardship adding to the reward of having dragged myself through the distance.

MARATHON 9: 4ᵀᴴ JUNE 2012

What a difference a day makes! I surprised myself with how I felt like I was resetting each morning. It was unbelievable. I was just physically and mentally beaten after each unrelenting day. I had come to master putting each marathon behind me, though. Once I crossed the day's finish line, I left my work in the office, no matter how tough a day it was on the concrete. I switched my attention to repairing my damaged body, enjoying my friends' company in our new surroundings and cherishing the warm, locally supplied calories. There was no energy wasted rehashing the day's torture or worrying about tomorrow's challenges.

Except for the torture in the middle of night four, I was sleeping the best I'd ever slept. Probably no surprise, given the toll I forced upon my body. Regardless of the toll, I was jumping out of bed each morning bright-eyed and bushy-tailed, seconds before my alarm, like I was about to jet off on a holiday I'd saved all year for, raring to get going. I couldn't put my finger on why it was so much easier now than regularly having to drag myself out of bed during training. Maybe the run's positive impact was more tangible as I saw euros getting donated as the dashed line on the map got filled in, slowly but surely. Maybe living your dream just makes you feel this way – alive, engaged and energised. Each day started with a clean slate. Each day a little further and a little more money raised, filling me with a sense of purpose. If only I could put this feeling in a bottle and sell it, I'd be a billionaire.

The sun was back out, which is always a help with the mood. I settled into a comfortable pace without any strappings on my body for a nice change. My quad strain, which the physio told me to rest for four days, wasn't troubling me at all today. I didn't understand it, but I certainly was not complaining. The disappearance of this injury added immensely to the day's good vibes.

The only problems during day nine crept in around the 12-kilometre mark. My Achilles tendon began feeling tender and was making an unpleasant clicking noise when I stretched it. Learning from past mistakes, I eased off the pace, trying to minimise aggravation as much as possible. The target of 35 marathons was firmly on my mind, and despite feeling relatively pain-free in comparison to the past week, I wasn't going to get ahead of myself and overcook it. I had to be smart and keep plenty in reserve.

Things were going well, with a flat route into Belfast limiting the stress and damage to my Achilles. I would have loved some physio, but the Queen's celebration was still ruining prospects of treatment. To my surprise and joy, I took a whopping 50 minutes off the previous day's time and felt a million times better. Five hours and 4 minutes. Only day one was faster.

What a roller coaster this was turning out to be. All emotions felt magnified, the pain, frustration and the joy and pleasure. When we arrived in the city, there was a press guy there to take pictures of us. With that swiftly out of the way, we were off to the hotel. Unfortunately, it had fallen through for some reason. Off we went walking door to door to try to find a place to take us in. As ever, it was down to persistence. After two rejections we arrived at Jury's Inn in the city centre. They were only too delighted to come to the rescue. Third time lucky.

Given how the day went overall and with running to Belfast being a milestone of mine, I sniffed out a cosy snug and enjoyed a well-earned pint with Tom and Sean. The icing on the day's cake was the visit from my parents, who had driven all the way up from Waterford to spend time with me. After savouring the one lip-licking pint, I left the men in the pub and went to meet Mam and Dad. I was on cloud nine, and they were delighted to see me in such great spirits, walking the walk. More importantly, Mam was just relieved I was still in one piece. *It's as well she visited today*, I thought.

At 10:00 p.m., it was time for me to roll in. I was bunking with Tom and Sean, but there was still no sign of them. Half of me was happy they were enjoying their downtime, and the other half dreaded a 04:00 a.m. wake up by two bulls in a china shop. *Tomorrow should be ... interesting!*

MARATHON 10: 5TH JUNE 2012

The alarm sounded at its usual time of 07:00 a.m. I reached to my bedside table for my litre bottle of water to start hydrating myself. This morning it had vanished. *The lads must have been thirsty.* Although an inconvenience to the routine, I couldn't be annoyed. After hours of drinking, they somehow managed not to wake me up stumbling in. With that impressive accomplishment, the lack of water could slide. They probably did bash into everything, my comatose slumber too deep to be disturbed. Having got me as far as they had, I was glad they let their hair down and were enjoying the trip, although it wouldn't look like they were today. They were in deep hangover territory. Fragile, doesn't even come close. If I wasn't on my tenth marathon in as many days, I might have felt sorry for them.

The streets were eerily quiet for a weekday morning in the city centre. It seems Tom and Sean weren't the only ones making use of the Queen's Jubilee. My parents were there to meet us at today's start line, laughing at the groggy heads on the lads. Since it was nearby, Dad was mad to get a photo outside the 'South Belfast Northern Ireland Supporters Club' building before I set off. Mam rolled her eyes with a smile, 'Football on the brain!'

I headed towards Antrim, through Templepatrick. On my way there, I saw the support car pulled up with the passenger door open, Sean's head hanging out of it.

'I'm not going to be much use to you today, Al,' he struggled, trying to avoid eye contact with his puddle of puke.

Seeing the guys dying, I was glad I had the restraint to only have the one celebratory pint before leaving them. Although it was their own doing, they were up early, and we hit the road on time. Credit where credit was due, I'm sure steering and feeding me was the last thing they wanted to be doing.

I was hoping to build off yesterday's much-improved run but no luck. I was in decent shape and enjoying the run until kilometre 24, when my right hamstring flared up, along with the left Achilles tendon. It looked like every single body part would take a hammering at some stage along this journey. I rested by the roadside for a minute, cautiously stretching the most damaged parts and applying anti-inflammatory cream. This is what I signed up for. Can I take the punishment and keep moving forward?

My bleary-eyed team sent me the wrong way again, this time as we were passing through Antrim. The previous navigational blunders could be overcome quickly, taking the next immediate turn, not impacting the expected finish point by much. Today's cock-up put me out by over two kilometres, and it bothered me way more than it should. With only my thoughts to accompany me on the road, the negativity spiralled. *One wrong turn, fair enough, but how many more?* We were starting to clock them up since Dublin. The route was calculated around Ireland, joining dots 42.2 kilometres apart, each day stopping when the GPS watch struck the marathon distance. Granted, repeated wrong turns wouldn't impact the completion of 35 x 42.2-kilometre runs. Still, I was starting to think the accumulated errors would only land me in Cork on the final day of the challenge, over 100 kilometres shy of the Waterford City finish line. What would I do then? Have to abandon the dream of running the lap and drive to the Waterford Viking Marathon?

With disproportionate highs, came disproportionate lows, emotions magnified due to the challenge's extreme nature. I was fed up and pissed off from the wrong turn onwards. My mindset of focusing on the problem meant I made the run miserable for myself. As I was festering in my own negativity, the support car pulled up alongside.

'We've been trying all day but can't get any physios. The Queen's thing is still dragging on, sorry Al.'

Not only was I making enemies with the team in my head for a meagre wrong turn but I was now taking aim at the Queen. *It's a Tuesday! How is it still a Bank Holiday? She's been at this craic since Saturday!* Since entering Northern Ireland, I'd had no physio. None on Sunday, Monday and now none on Tuesday either. My coping mechanism of having a reward to look forward to at the finish line was taken from me again. The further bad news was feeding my downward mental trajectory. Not even the thought of double desserts would lift my mood on this occasion.

From kilometre 32, the injuries and frustrations were growing. Negative self-talk took over, and my hamstring felt like it could tear at any moment. *Fuckin' four-day bank holiday. No physio again. Bloody wrong turn. That's because they were on the sauce. Ugh, me hamstring is fucked.* It's draining just writing these kinds of thoughts, never mind having them on repeat whilst running a marathon on a wet and dreary Irish summer's day.

Life was made easier by the presence of my parents. They'd

drive up to me every so often and ask if I was okay or if I needed anything. I'd just be a dickhead to get onto Tom and Sean for the misdirection. They were friends giving up their time for free to see me achieve my dream. The internalised frustrations were doing me no good either. Unfortunately for my parents, they'd have to listen to me moaning and unloading about wrong turns, the Queen's Jubilee scuppering yet another physio session and this being sore and that being sore. As stupid as my woes were, just talking about it and being listened to relieved some of the annoyance.

After ranting and confiding in Mam and Dad, I just went on autopilot mode and gritted my teeth, alternating between walking and jogging forward. Entering Kells, I was counting down the kilometres to the finish line. *Three kilometres to go.* I'd keep glancing at the numbers on my watch, willing them to the marathon distance. *Two kilometres to go. It's in the bag. One kilometre to go. Finally.* Then I was done.

'That's it here, lads. It's a wrap. Thank fuck.'

We weren't able to spray-paint a marker on the road since the day ended on someone's doorstep. As usual, though, we took plenty of photos of the surroundings and marked it on a map, so we knew where to return to for the next marathon.

We drove immediately to the hotel, silence in the car, Tom and Sean hungover and sleep-deprived; me, an exhausted, grumpy fart. The hotel had sponsored two rooms. My own space felt so luxurious after the day's battle and the last few days of bunking in together. I went straight for an ice bath followed by a pleasurable warm shower, accelerating the decompression process. My parents treated us to lunch in the hotel, saving us from leaving in search of a sponsored meal and helping dampen the atmosphere of exhaustion. Starter, mains, dessert and a jug of water; I was myself again, smiling once more.

With the recovery protocol followed and feeling 100 times better, it was time to plug in my GPS watch to upload the day's marathon and update the blog.

'SHIT! 41.2 kilometres!'

I rubbed my eyes and looked again.

'That can't be? Yep. Fuckin' idiot.' Amidst the day's distractions, I'd been counting down to the wrong number and had stopped one kilometre short of the marathon.

I went straight to Tom and Sean's door to break the news. The meal and shower didn't seem to have had the same rejuvenating effect on them, both men dressed down and ready for a pre-dinner siesta.

'Sorry guys, I fucked up. I still have one kilometre left to run. I stopped too early like an idiot. I can't count.'

'You're kidding?'

I showed them the watch to remove any doubt and make sure I didn't just imagine it.

'Can you just run an extra kilometre tomorrow?'

'Can't. It's a marathon a day, so 41.2 kilometres today and 43.2 kilometres tomorrow won't cut it.'

This was a kick in the teeth to all of us after what felt like our longest day, but we just had to get on with it. It was no Guinness World Record, and nothing was stopping me from making up the distance the next day, as Sean suggested, but it didn't line up with my values of staying true to my original rules. Tom drove us back to the finish marker, where I'd stopped about two hours earlier. I just laughed the error off, feeling in a completely different mental space than a few hours previous. Rather than stay in the comfy hotel and catch up on missed sleep, Sean laced up his runners, and DJ Tom got the music flowing. The kilometre felt like nothing, primarily down to the team's attitude, making light of the situation – Sean mooning his arse to Tom, as Tom tried to record my stupid mistake on camera. We may not have been a professional Dean Karnazes outfit, but the three Irish novices on a shoestring were sure as hell making ground. Combining my two runs from the day, I'd completed the marathon distance in 5 hours and 35 minutes. Four hundred and twenty-two kilometres completed in 10 days! *Yes boy.*

MARATHON 11: 6ᵀᴴ JUNE 2012

It was a concerning start to the day, waking up with some kind of rash on my chin. The stress and demands of the physical challenge were now visible on my face. After going through years of acne and pushing through a world of pain to run this far, a stinging face was nothing. I shrugged it off and made a mental note to monitor it.

Having watched me and joined me for a few kilometres on previous days and having bounced back from the mother of all hangovers, Sean was intrigued to give a full marathon a go. There was only one turn required today – towards Ballycastle, accommodation was in place and, thank Christ, we had a physio booked too. With logistics looked after, I was glad of Sean's company on the concrete, allowing me a nice holiday from the voice in my head. There was also a sense of satisfaction helping Sean take a leap towards his first marathon, far beyond his comfort zone, which generally consisted of going for an odd five-kilometre jog now and then.

The plan of action was to get to Ballycastle on the north-east coast in as close to one piece as possible. With my body still deteriorating and the team still heading north – away from home, I played it safe, running roughly one kilometre and taking a short walking breather. My right quad, knees and left Achilles were all causing me bother from the start. I had to walk a fine line. I knew I was never going to cover the entire route pain-free. I'd just have to continue to absorb the punishment but not push to the extent that I couldn't put one foot in front of the other – pain but not too much pain. I had to be patient and sensible and learn when to take my foot off the gas a fraction, to ensure I lived to fight another day, and another day, and another day. *Just get to the physio*, was the mantra on this day's marathon. Just knowing I could have treatment after this marathon put a pep in my step, with my body not having got any attention over the last three days.

The A26 and A44 were the dodgiest roads I'd run on to date. This says a lot since I'd already run on a motorway and through Dublin City Centre. The hard shoulder was non-existent for large stretches of the route, making for uneasy and treacherous running conditions. The dual carriageway was a heavily used stretch, and a lot of the speeding traffic consisted of large articulated lorries, increasing the fear factor. It was the first time traffic gave me grave cause for concern, each piece of roadkill I passed creating a more and more ominous atmosphere. Even though it was clear daylight, with no fog or rain impeding visibility, we gave the elevated lorry drivers the benefit of the doubt.

'Maybe they can't see us. That's why they're not slowing down or indicating around us.'

We only had the one hi-vis vest since I hadn't anticipated anyone wanting to put themselves through this ordeal with me. Sean suggested we implement 'Operation Get Behind Sean', whereby he'd wear the yellow hi-vis vest, and I'd cower behind him.

'If they hit me, they'll have slowed down a fraction by the time they run you over, and you might get away with continuing the run,' Sean joked darkly.

We either had to stop and re-route or make light of a bad situation while proceeding with caution. We chose the latter. The reflective vest turned out to be ineffective, and it didn't make a blind bit of difference to the driver's speed or the reckless proximity with which they flew past our petrified faces. I'm not sure what was going on in their heads, as lorry drivers nearly turned us to mush on numerous occasions. The reward for roaring past at breakneck speeds, within inches of us, was that they would save 10 seconds on their journey. The risk was they'd kill two charity runners. They were probably thinking, *what are these two twats doing on my haulage road? Not on my watch.* After a few too many close shaves; unable to influence driver behaviour, we controlled what we could, stopping and jumping off to the side of the road each time oncoming traffic came hurtling toward us.

Veering to safety from vehicles, brought its own less

apparent risks. With all my focus on the oncoming traffic, I took my eye off the uneven ground which dropped off steeply. I rolled over on my ankle with my body quickly following and ended up in a heap on the ground. Rolling with it, thankfully, prevented severe damage. As a heap on the concrete, I sighed relief. I couldn't afford to break or sprain an ankle with more than 24 marathons left ahead of me. I had to switch to focusing on two threats now, which drew additional fuel from the already overworked battery.

Having to worry about speeding traffic on one side and foot placement on the other certainly didn't make for comfortable running, let alone enjoyable running. Thinking of my first marathon experience in Dublin, I felt so bad for Sean. Pretty grim stuff. Luckily, Sean's attitude was lively positivity and we joked and laughed our way through the inherent dangers.

Traffic quietened a bit, and the road narrowed as we took our one turn for the day towards the northern coastline of Ballycastle, via Armoy. Although the dual carriageway had stopped, the A44 was a long straight, unobstructed road, which meant drivers continued to act like they were in the World Rally Championships. The continuous green farmland which surrounded us on both sides was a pleasant distraction, but we couldn't risk letting our guards down much to take in the beauty.

Sean did really well over the distance although I could see he'd have preferred to keep the pace constant, rather than turning up and down the dial to allow some relief for my knees and mind. This section of the road won my title of 'the most dangerous marathon'. It took 5 hours and 47 minutes, a bit slower than the previous marathon. Still, I made it to the physio without incurring too much more damage, and we didn't get hit by a moving vehicle – great success.

With the marathon done, I advised Sean he wasn't done yet. 'If you want the full experience and want to try reduce tomorrow's aches, you'll need an ice bath. I have it running for you.'

Usually, I sit in the empty bath and turn the cold tap on, adding ice once my legs are submerged. Then I get the 10-minute timer going. This tactic allows the body to slowly acclimatise to the freezing temperature and there's no drastic shock to the system, wincing, or gasping for air. I thought it would be funnier for Tom and me to withhold that information from Sean, fill her up and leave the ice to sit for a while, dropping the temperature another degree or two.

'Sean, your lovely bath's ready dear!'

The face of terror and the squeals coming out of a grown man were priceless, as he ungracefully broke the water's surface, fighting the internal voice that was now audible in the neighbour's house.

'Why am I doing this?! It's not funny! Help, you cruel bastards!'

MARATHON 12: 7TH JUNE 2012

Day 12 saw me achieve a personal worst marathon of 6 hours and 34 minutes – a long aul' slog of a day. After assessing the damage to my body, the previous day's physio had advised me to walk up hills, rather than run. The hope was that this would reduce the throbbing of my Achilles tendon. My hamstring was feeling the distance too, so it was bandaged up for good measure.

I never got going with so many hills in front of me. I'd get running at a steady pace but would have to break the rhythm to walk the hills. I found myself trying to make up for lost time then, accelerating back to a run. I'd have to remind myself to slow down. Just as I found a sensible pace, it would be time for another hill, forcing a repeat of the frustrating process.

The route levelled out around the 12-kilometre mark when I was fully warmed up and able to eventually enjoy five kilometres in this gorgeous landscape. Open green fields continued to my left, as the greenery to my right transitioned into a rugged rockface, exposed by the Atlantic's power.

It was a life in extremes, condensed into a 42.2-kilometre journey. Although I grew accustomed to my crazy daily routine, nothing ever felt mundane, and I never felt so alive. The agony required focus from my mind to persevere. Whenever the haze of energy-zapping suffering lifted, mental space became available to appreciate my surroundings and my fortunate circumstances. I was outside, roaming Ireland's landscapes, grateful for the lull in pain. I felt more than just gratitude in scenery like this, I was euphoric, deeply inhaling the countryside. I was engaged in a passion project for a meaningful cause, with my friends and family supporting me, travelling on foot through a postcard landscape. I went through an overwhelming pendulum of emotions, from cursing my Achilles and the barrage of hills to feeling like I wouldn't want to be anywhere else in the world. And I'd only reached kilometre 17!

There are good days and bad days in life – most days

fly by without anything of note worth storing to memory. We get clobbered by loss and suffering, begging for the return of mundanity, which comes in time, and then we are lifted with love or joy, all to be repeated in no specific sequence. The 12 days so far had been an amplified version of life without any mundanity in between. The concentration of feelings and emotions was a hell of a whirlwind.

My gaze left the wild Atlantic and returned to an imminent hill. I slowed to a walk as instructed and took it in my stride. Breaking the crest of the hill, I went running again. *Shit! Ah!* I experienced a shot of pain like a nail being hammered into the front of my right knee, forcing me to stop abruptly. It was like nothing I'd experienced before. *Fuck, let's just walk for a minute, relax yourself.* I couldn't relax. For all the pain I knew I could take, the jarring knee pain was not something to simply run off.

Walking returned my body to a steady but bearable drip of discomfort that I'd become accustomed to. The walk became boring after a few minutes. I decided it was time to try running since no noteworthy signals were sent from my knee since starting to stroll. *Maybe it was a once-off.* I pushed off to a jog again. *Nope, that was worse. Shite, this is not good.* Not one to give up on an idea too quickly, I thought it was worth at least trying to persevere through it. After another few minutes walking, I gave the jogging one more right go but was welcomed with the same sharp dose of pain, my body instinctively pulling back. My mind had other plans. On the first and second attempt, I gave up after just one stride. *Let's try 50 metres,* I thought. I wanted to push it, but the feeling was too intense, and I had to stop after only three strides.

'Fuckity fuck fuck!'

Having failed repeatedly, I had no choice but to admit defeat. It was time to adapt and overcome.

'Lads!? I'm going to have to walk the rest of this one. My knee's banjaxed. At this stage, we won't have time to visit the Giant's Causeway. Sorry, men. Was really looking forward to it and all.' I was sickened. The Giant's Causeway and the Cliffs of Moher were the only landmarks I'd set out as must-visits since we were due to pass right by them. I hadn't time to see them when driving the route with Dad either, as we had been against the clock.

To fit the mood, the clouds rolled in, and it began pissing rain. If this wasn't the bottom, it was pretty damn close – injured, unable to run, miserable weather, half-marathon left today and another 23 marathons after that. You can take things for granted until they're entirely taken from you. The intermittent jog-the-flats-and-walk-the-hills approach had been soul-destroying but now, not even able for that, I was yearning for the ability to jog even 10 metres.

Slowed to a walk, the rain soaked me to the bone. I was misery personified. Slowly sploshing forward, I thought continually about my knee and what that meant for the challenge: this was punishment, but I wasn't going to surrender. The route took me through an officially designated 'Area of Outstanding Natural Beauty', a predominantly coastal road, with fields, the sea and cliff edges – but I was uninterested at this point. I made a mental note to return when I could enjoy the beauty but, for now, my hood was up, my head was down, and my blinkers only allowed me to take in the next step. I had to strip the challenge right back to one step at a time.

Having strapped my knee up and walked for what felt like an eternity, I was able to run intermittently again as I came into Portrush. I consciously shortened my stride, to not overstretch my knee. I was vigilant for any signs of increased pain, sure to walk at the first sign of a red flag being raised.

With no piercing pain, my gaze lifted from the next step to the next signpost. I never allowed myself to get overawed by the challenge. When things started to feel like too much, I just pulled the task within arm's length to cope with the difficulty. Not 35 marathons. Not one marathon. Sometimes, just a step at a time, a kilometre at a time, five minutes at a time or one landmark at a time. It varied, but the approach was the same – make it bite-sized and forget about the meal's size.

The day dragged, and I was fed up with bananas and gels, particularly since I could not run and exert myself. Proper nutrition wasn't hitting the spot. I was cold, wet, sore and annoyed. I craved filth and listened to my body. 'Would you mind getting me something in a deli or take away, lads? I can't be arsed with Jaffa Cakes and fruit on a shitty day like this.'

'Any preference?'

'Anything as long as it's warm and tasty looking.'

That day, I believe I became the first person to devour a sausage burger bun combo during a marathon, which gave me great joy and confused the lads!

'You're a gas man! So, you run 12 marathons in 12 days,

and you're like, "Yeah, whatever!" but you eat a burger during one, and you're like a proud child? You've got strange measures of success, Alo,' they laughed. It was another one down, a notable one, one-third of the way around the island and now heading west, instead of north.

MARATHON 13: 8TH JUNE 2012

After just one day off, Sean was on board for another marathon today.

'Some man for one man!' I told him.

I was astonished, recalling the disabled state of my body after my first marathon. I couldn't walk to class two days later, never mind contemplate covering another 42.2 kilometres. He was making me look like a right lightweight. I loved it. Nutter!

The lads' attitudes were everything. They kept the mood light at all times, mostly taking the piss out of me. We were just three Irish men on a road trip, having the craic – one a little less craic than the others but I was enjoying myself, nonetheless. Bar the few forgivable wrong turns, these acting tour managers were on top of their game and going above and beyond to make my life as easy as possible in the circumstance. It was such a weight off, not having to give a thought to the logistics again. They made it so I just had to show up and run, not having to attend another meeting, make another call or send another email.

The previous marathon had been my longest day and the most worrying, as far as my body was concerned. Gradual, slowly deteriorating injuries were one thing to soak up, but the penetrating pain in my knee was just next level – not a sensation to risk pushing through. The knee trouble had been day 12. Day 13 was a new day and a fresh start. Maybe I'd have to have the same struggle, perhaps a new struggle. I hoped for peace and no battles, but I was ready for war if it came to it.

08:30 a.m. on the button and a wet and windy run from Coleraine began. My Achilles was taped up to the nines in an attempt to protect it. Unsurprisingly my knee was the primary source of tenderness at the start.

As the marathon progressed, my knee was somehow starting to feel better and better. Just so I didn't get too carried away, my Achilles was getting worse and worse. I had to laugh. By now, I just accepted my body's ever-changing response to the demands I was putting on it. It made little sense that I'd strain a muscle after running a marathon, I'd run another marathon, and it would be worse, but by the next marathon, the muscle strain had disappeared. I just accepted something is always going to be hurting, and my body is doing a great job at healing itself, just in its own time and not all at once. It didn't have to make sense, and I didn't need to understand it, I just had to keep constant forward motion.

My suffering had some company. Sean, who breezed his first marathon two days ago, was having second thoughts as we ran towards Derry.

'Is it smart to be doing this again after one day's rest?' Sean asked.

'God no! You're as thick as me, if not worse. I was stupid enough to do a marathon untrained, but I at least had the sense not to move for three days after it. You're on another level!'

He was hurting, and the hardship was visible in his demeanour. No wonder. I encouraged him along, and in return, he encouraged me. There were no medals, crowds, prize money or social media platforms to update, just him quietly proving something to himself. I took great inspiration from him.

We were two miserable sods, slowly plodding through the rain, drenched, having to endure Tom being smug in the car.

'What's the holdup, eh? Why so slow? I better turn down this heating it's getting too warm in here.'

'Fuck off Tom and leave me alone!' Sean shouted with a smile.

Tom blasted Bill Withers 'Use Me' in retaliation, giving poor Sean a taste of his own medicine, now not enjoying the sounds as much, given the beating his body was taking. It was a slow wet laboured day, clocking a time of 6 hours and 9 minutes, landing us just east of Derry. Taking some positives, Sean got the job done, I was faster than the previous day, and the pain stayed at bearable levels throughout, with no repeat alarm bells.

Reaching the physio, they told me that I had Achilles tendonitis, which would make life problematic for the remainder of the challenge.

'If you had any sense, you'd rest it completely, but since you've run this far already, I'd imagine sense isn't a strong point.'

'No, not at all. No days' rest. Them's the rules!'

After a relaxing light rub-down, I got the opportunity to use a cryotherapy pool filled with water at a bitter 2°C. The Irish sea in the summer is around 15°C, so this was bloody cold. Anything was worth a try to reduce the inflammation and potentially ease the suffering.

MARATHON 14: 9ᵀᴴ JUNE 2012

The challenge was not getting any easier as the days accumulated, as evidenced by my marathon times. This morning was a struggle; I was not feeling reinvigorated like previous mornings. It felt like an immediate continuation of my previous marathon: kilometre number 43.

Although my energy levels were down, there was a vast improvement in my Achilles. It retreated to a manageable 2/10 pain, instead of 8/10. In an attempt to override the lag in energy levels, I stuffed my face with a gel, banana and Jaffa Cakes at kilometre six, tripling my regular intake at this juncture. In training, food seemed to resolve any lethargic feelings, and I thought it better to overdo it than underdo it.

Finding things harder than usual, for the first time I asked Tom and Sean for moral support, seeing if either would join me on the bicycle after the kilometre six pit stop. We negotiated our way through the historic streets of Derry together. By kilometre 14, I was out of the rut with the help of sugar and friends, back solo running again. This was a new challenge, having the script flipped, fighting to overcome adversity during the first portion of the marathon rather than facing the beast towards the mid to latter half.

With my physical and mental state on an upward trajectory, I perked up even more crossing the next personal milestone: departing Northern Ireland and returning to the Republic. Another small moment to mark progress and take some pleasure from.

With everything turning for the better, the men wanted a break from babysitting me. They pulled up beside me with the window rolled down and looked like giddy schoolgirls.

'What's up? All good?' I asked.

'You won't believe it! We saw a sign for a town called *Muff*! We need to visit!'

I don't think I'd seen them this enthused the whole trip. Who was I to deny the joy visible on these young faces, when faced with the opportunity to visit Muff?

'Go enjoy yourselves and take some pictures. I'm on this road 'til the finish, so you know where to find me. Have fun!'

Most of the photographic evidence of this marathon consists of the support team 10 kilometres off the route, next to the town's signposts, 'Muff', 'Welcome to Muff', 'Muff Welcomes You' and 'The Squealin' Pig Muff' pub. You got to enjoy and laugh at life's simple pleasures, haven't you?

In stark contrast to the lad's silly immature excitement, I ran past more than five plaques along the roadside, commemorating those that died in traffic accidents on the stretch from Derry to Letterkenny. Left on my own, with the solitude of my thoughts, I appreciated how lucky I was to be alive and healthy, able to move freely and try to do some good. I felt I was right where I should be, grabbing hold of life and pushing the limits with purpose.

Kilometre 29 saw me come to an abrupt stop, with the unpleasant yet now familiar sensation in my knee. *Not again. Give me a break. Fuck sake!*

I was reminded of a Martin Luther King line, 'If you can't run, walk. If you can't walk, crawl, but by all means, keep moving.'

Walk, Al. Just keep going, a step at a time, I told myself.

As with the day on the Causeway Coast, I allowed myself some respite before restarting the engines. On this occasion, my body cut me some slack, and my knee permitted me to return to a cautious run after some persistent attempts. Five hours and 56 minutes were chalked on the scoreboard, and another marathon was in the bag.

EIGHT

TURNING THE CORNER

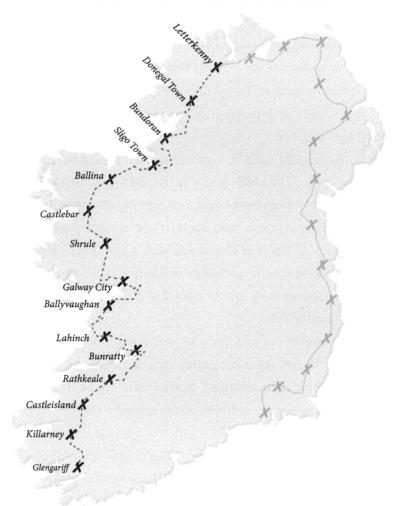

DAY 15 - DAY 28:
Letterkenny–Donegal Town–Bundoran–Sligo Town–Ballina–
Castlebar–Shrule–Galway City–Ballyvaughan–Lahinch–
Bunratty–Rathkeale–Castleisland–Killarney–Glengariff

MARATHON 15: 10TH JUNE 2012

Feeling the accumulating damage, I went to bed even earlier than usual, hoping sleep would work its magic. I conked out for over 10 hours and felt all the better in the morning for the smart move.

We made our way out of Letterkenny, completing the northern section of the journey, turning south for the next 13 days: another small milestone to take some satisfaction from.

'You've run up the country and across it. All downhill now, boy,' the lads joked.

Exiting the town, I found myself on a steep back road, regretting the route I had chosen but embracing the beauty of it. The narrow road was free of road markings, capable of taking just a car at a time, although there was no traffic in the serene setting. Hedgerows and trees lined either side, with green grass stretching beyond, dotted with large mature tree canopies. I laboured my way upwards, working for the reward of a better vantage point over the countryside.

'I thought you said it was all feckin' downhill! Ugh! Not a bad view, though, eh?' After getting off to a positive start, things slowed towards kilometre 14 as I decided to walk a few of the hills, protecting my injured Achilles, which was now the bane of my life.

I was back in my stride running through Ballybofey, towards Donegal Town, as temperatures reached the 20s. As the marathon progressed, I was growing stronger. The aching was subsiding as I returned to my quicker training pace for a stint. The warm rays on my face and a light breeze in my hair, along with the speed and subdued pain levels, brought back fond memories of roaming around the trails of the Phoenix Park. The nostalgia brought a smile to my face, thinking of the journey from training novice to here.

The cherry on top was the spectacular scenery. Moving towards Donegal Town, we passed Lough Mourne, running into Barnesmore Gap mountain pass. Down in the valley, a shallow stream flowed along the roadside and we stopped to wet our feet amidst the impressive landscape. The Bluestack Mountains rose either side of the pass, conifer woods making it resemble Canada, but this was our beautiful Ireland.

If only all the runs felt like the last nine kilometres, I thought. Then again, would there be true satisfaction if it all felt like sunshine? I don't think so. The days that pain was edging to the brink and cold rain pelted my face were the days that were the test; the days I had to force myself to break a glass ceiling and step beyond my imagined limitations. Anyone could run well when rested on a sunny summer's day but, to steal a Franklin D. Roosevelt line, 'a smooth sea never made a skilled sailor.' I wanted to enter the eye of the storm and conquer it, coming out the other side battle-tested and more capable than when I entered.

That said, I would enjoy the fair-weather sailing when it presented itself. Today was 10 minutes quicker than the last marathon, finishing in a time of 5 hours and 44 minutes.

MARATHON 16: 11TH JUNE 2012

The first nine kilometres into Donegal Town flew by, and I picked up where I had left off, high on life. I got encouragement from a cyclist who whizzed past me on the way into Ballyshannon. I highly doubt they knew the extent of what I was up to. They just saw me running and said, 'Keep it up, big man.' Everything on this challenge was intensified, and the kind words from a passing stranger made my day, especially in light of only tipping over the €5,000 mark – still €30,000 short of my target. It just goes to show a simple bit of encouragement or kindness can have a profound impact on somebody, making an unbearable day bearable or a good day even better.

After the unexpected gee up, I enjoyed some quick kilometres breaking through the 30-kilometre marker, 'quick' being a relative term!

Coming into Bundoran, I was getting a bit distracted, having the craic with the lads, stopping to look at this and that and petting a roadside donkey. *Get this marathon done*, I reminded myself. Feeling good, I put the foot down, but my body reminded me of my limitations with a sharp pain in my right heel.

'Ow! That's a new one.'

Don't be a tit. I slowed to a sensible pace once more for the last kilometre or two. Still, I knocked another 10 minutes off the previous marathon, which had already been 10 minutes off the marathon before that, which was about 10 minutes faster than the marathon before that. My trajectory was improving as my body seemed to adapt finally.

Finishing near the sea, I wanted a break from the ice baths for the natural elixir. The sea was a concerning shade of poo, so we decided to keep the jumpers on and just get the legs covered, not wanting to risk putting our heads anywhere near the surface of the water.

'Lads, how grim is this water, it looks ...' said Sean, as he slipped on a rock and submerged himself with a splash, t-shirt, hoody and all! Once again, Tom and I could enjoy a laugh at the expense of Sean and his traumatic ice bath experiences.

MARATHON 17: 12ᵀᴴ JUNE 2012

When my body and times were deteriorating, I always reminded myself tomorrow was a fresh start and could be better. I kept hope. When things were going well, and I was going from strength to strength, I never thought the day could be a banana skin that would be my demise. My eternal optimism sometimes left me thinking I'd get stronger and faster, with less and less pain. This hopefulness left me somewhat flat-footed when a storm steamrolled in.

Nearing the midway point of the five-week challenge, my pilgrimage from Bundoran to Sligo was my most testing day of the lot.

Sean, the hero, was on for yet another marathon run.

'Do you mind if I join you again?'

'Another one? You feeling up for it?'

'It's my last day – why not go for three and end on a high note?'

'Go on, ya good thing! No arguments from me if you're game. Glad to have you, bud.'

Tom was a certified tour manager by now, so we left him to his own devices in the Nissan headquarters as Sean and I laced up and got to work.

For the first 16 kilometres, we chatted away casually,

enjoying the views of the mountains and covering the entire Leitrim coastline – all four kilometres – with ease! The Irish landscapes often left me in awe, exceeding my expectations when I initially aspired to see the country on foot. The mighty Benbulbin came in to view, protruding dramatically from the surrounding countryside. The flat-topped green mountain gives Australia's dusty red Uluru a run for its money, in my book.

The beauty of travelling by foot along this tourist trail came at a steep price. My left Achilles tendon was now screaming, like someone was grabbing it with the full force of their grip, with a piercing pain each time my foot struck the ground. You might have surmised at this stage that I've got a high pain tolerance. Despite this, I was making scrunched grimacing facial expressions and audible grunts even when walking. The hurt wasn't helped by the hills which made running impossible for me; the pain stopping just shy of unbearable with the inclines torturing my heel.

'Did you ever feel like quitting or have any doubts about your ability to see the challenge through to the end?' I was often asked. The honest short answer is no. Not even in the agony of this day, did I think I would not finish the day's distance and all the remaining marathons. It wasn't because I thought I was some great runner: far from it, as evidenced by my unimpressive marathon times and short training duration. I was mentally unstoppable because I had never felt so committed and passionate about something in my entire life. I had been obsessed with the challenge since March 2011. I'd invested too much of myself into the development process. The memories of young fallen friends drove me to persevere; the dark emotions of Dad's near-death experience fuelling me through the difficulty. I had the confidence from completing all the hours upon hours of solitary road and trail runs, gym sessions, meetings, phone calls and emails. For me not to finish, I'd have had to be hospitalised and unable to make any forward movement. Until then, I was unwilling to relent. I was in agony, yes, but this temporary physical suffering was bearable in the context of what I'd endured up to this point.

I wasn't thinking about further studies or a career or anything else bar the present moment and my good fortune in having the opportunity and ability to do what I was doing. I had no real responsibility with dependents or a mortgage, no money to my name, and was hurting daily, but I'd never felt so fulfilled. I was revelling in the outdoor surroundings and the new challenges that tried to stop me but failed time and time again, each victory adding another wafer-thin layer to my armour.

Unable to run the inclines, I was reduced to walking large sections of the day, significantly slowing progress. I hobbled and cursed my way along the route from the 16-kilometre mark onwards. I wasn't alone in my suffering; Sean was in a tough spot too. Usually wired to the moon, his third marathon in the space of a week was hitting him hard. The strain of the day was enough to quieten us both as we fought our fights.

At kilometre 30, Aisling Kennedy, my friend and neighbour, was dropped off by her boyfriend, Eddy, to join Tom in the support team. Eddy had driven Aisling up from Waterford to Sligo, a four-hour trek, with the plan to turn right around to crate Sean back home.

Because of the crippled state I was in, we were nowhere

near finishing within the time we hoped for. Eddy was in a rush back, which left Sean in a conundrum. Sean could stop the agony right away, jump in the car for a snooze and wake up at home four hours later. Or he could continue to take a beating for another 11 kilometres and then endure Ireland's public transport system, crammed on a bus via Dublin, taking some seven hours to crawl home. There was zero obligation for Sean to continue, and every reason to take the lift offered; 99% of people would have taken the opportunity to stop the suffering.

'What's it to be, Sean?'

'I'm staying here, Al. I've come through too much today to stop now. Don't want to leave you hanging on a tough one either. I might as well finish.'

Tom, Aisling and Eddy looked flabbergasted. I laughed and put my arm over his shoulder.

'Some eejit! Love it. Let's crack on then.'

We waved goodbye to Eddy and trudged onwards. We were both struggling. Some days it was ballerina slippers, graceful efficiency; some days it was boxing gloves, biting down on the gumshield, swinging wild fists. There were no questions about what kind of day this was.

I laughed when he agreed to stay, but all jokes aside, I drew massive inspiration from his actions and gained even more respect for him. He was a lively messer, his resilience taking me by surprise. He more than proved himself to be a tough cookie over the week. His commitment to himself, and to me and the challenge – as evidenced by his rejecting the easy exit – was powerfully motivating.

We must have looked a right pair, hobbling forward in focused silence, except for a few unsavoury words here and there when the pain couldn't be contained. Aisling, a psychiatric nurse, probably had an opinion or two formed within minutes of joining the crew. We thought it best not to ask for her professional judgment.

On this most difficult of days for my body, my mind worked overtime as I visualised hugging my family at the finish line and handing fat cheques to the charities with my dad. These mental images would buy me another kilometre or two. That was all I needed, and boy was I glad to see my watch tick to 42.2 kilometres and to stop moving. There were hugs all around after this one. Tom was kind enough to lend me a shoulder of support to get me to the car and then drove poor Sean to the bus station. I pitied the unfortunate souls who had to sit beside him; he hadn't had time to shower after the 6 hours and 25 minutes of battling.

With Sean dropped off, I collapsed across the back seat of the car in silence, broken. I shimmied to my hotel room, Aisling and Tom helping haul my luggage as I huffed and puffed under my own body weight. Once the regular ice bath was complete, I plonked to the floor of the shower with my head in my hands and let the warm water soothe my defeated mind and body.

To further mark the occasion of the grimmest marathon to date, my first toenail came off. I could finally call myself an official ultra-distance runner, earning the last of my stripes. This one had eluded me thus far as I'd ticked off hitting the wall, thigh chafing, raw nipples, blisters, blackened toenails and every muscle, tendon and joint ache there was.

The foot swelling experienced over the first five or so days had subsided, along with the general foot aches, as my body toughened to fulfil its new role. The blisters didn't relent. Despite never suffering any blisters before day two, they would inevitably persist once they began, given I had soggy runners on rainy days and sweaty runners on dry days. Some nasty oozing blisters formed beneath my toenails as my poor feet squeezed against the shoe with each stride. The liquid bubbles grew, and the constant trauma eventually forced the nail from my foot. There you go. One of the many joys of the challenge. Apologies if you were eating!

MARATHON 18: 13ᵀᴴ JUNE 2012

It was the most apprehensive I'd been so far. Every other day I had looked forward with hope and optimism, regardless of the highs or lows that went before. Because the previous day had been the most difficult, it was impossible to forget. While stretching, eating breakfast, and en route to the start, the hardship was on my mind. I disliked this unusual apprehensive feeling. Being anxious wasn't going to help anything. It was a drain of energy, but I couldn't shake it off.

My uncharacteristic worry subsided a little when we passed a group of secondary school students about to sit their Leaving Certificate exams. Now they looked anxious, and had more reason to be, with a lot perceived to be riding on the final exams. I felt like saying, *You've got nothing to worry about lads. You've done the work you could and whatever you know, you know, and what you don't, you don't. Worrying won't help you recall a thing. Even if things go totally tits up today, there are your other subjects, and there's next year or some workaround to get where you want.* It was somehow easier giving this imaginary advice to them, rather than talk to myself in a more supportive tone. I needed to step out of myself. I'd never coach me by saying, 'Yesterday was horrendous, and you'll probably suck again today,' which was where my mind was at that morning. Instead, I thought, *Yesterday is gone. Draw a line under it. Focus on what you're doing each kilometre today. Just concern yourself with moving your body forward to the next kilometre marker, and if you need to slow down, what harm?*

I learned that I needed to talk to myself as I would to others, with support, understanding, encouragement and positivity, bringing solutions and not just highlighting problems. Today's run was challenging, but the physical suffering wasn't a patch on yesterday's battle. My mind wasn't allowed space to think about the sensations pulsing through my pain receptors for most of the day, as there was clearly a more significant threat; I passed a shocking number of roadside memorials. I was acutely switched on to the oncoming traffic, which came far too close for comfort at times.

My Achilles was relatively subdued to begin with, gradually ratcheting up from a 2/10 to a notable 5/10 on my pain scale, around the mid-way point of the run. By kilometre 38, I had to walk gingerly as the pain dial was right back up to 10/10, where it had been most of the previous day. My heel was clinging on by a thread. The only silver lining was that the brutal pain was occurring much closer to the finish line: only four kilometres of torment.

If this wasn't enough, my hay fever reared its ugly head

again. I wanted to rip my eyes out. Often, when one part of the anatomy screams, it can be quickly forgotten if another problem crops up. Unfortunately, this didn't hold, on today's outing. The misery of pollen scouring my eyeballs did not take anything from the fire blazing in my heel. The circumstances at the end were extraordinarily grim; I was shuffling, only opening my eyes every few steps to get my bearings.

In agony, my heel was screaming and my eyes heavily bloodshot, I just about managed to walk the final three kilometres. It was another gloomy day at the office.

I scraped home in 5 hours and 58 minutes, officially crossing the half-way mark of the challenge but I was too battered to celebrate the achievement. I urgently needed medication for my eyes and ice for my roaring Achilles.

Mixing pain with pleasure, The Ice House Hotel, Ballina, generously put us up for the night. I looked a right mess arriving into the reception of this fine establishment, stinking and struggling to see and walk but the receptionist remained professional, welcoming me warmly.

I limped to my room, finding a smartly dressed employee on hand and offering to prepare my bath for me. I had to laugh. I was in a bad way and realised I had a look to match, catching my sad reflection in the bathroom mirror. Yet there I was like a king, having his bath readied for him.

'You're grand, I can manage the bath,' I told the man, feeling uncomfortable about being attended to with this high-level service.

'Not at all, sir, you can relax.'

'If you insist. Thanks, a mil.' *Oh, this is awkward …* 'Eh, I'm very sorry. Eh, not the hot tap, please. Would you mind just sticking on the cold one? Sorry for being contrary.'

It went from being awkward and strange for me, to be weird for both of us, in this odd bathroom scene.

'Just run the cold tap, sir?' he hesitated.

'Yeah, if that's alright. It's to help with my recovery from a long run I did today. Well, at least I'm told it helps.'

'No problem, sir. I guess you don't want the candles if it's not a relaxing bath?'

'Feck it. I'll spoil myself today. Work away with lighting the candles. Thanks.'

There was a knock on the door. Another well-groomed upright man arrived at the door with a silver Champagne bucket in hand and a neatly folded white cloth over his forearm.

'Good evening, sir. Your ice. Where would you like me to put it?'

'In there please,' pointing towards the bathroom.

I caught his perplexed look in the bathroom mirror, as he made eye contact with the lad lighting the candles, as the blue tap flooded into the tub. I felt obliged to justify my peculiarity to him too. The humour of the scenario was exactly what I needed to soften the gruelling day's harshness.

'Enjoy your bath?' they said as a question, rather than a statement, leaving me to my first ever candlelit ice bath. Bit of a waste really, since all I could do was close and vigorously rub my redraw eyelids, waiting for Aisling or Tom to come to my rescue with eye drops and antihistamine tablets.

Few things can compare to the generosity of a stranger. A man by the name of Alan Murphy called down to the boutique hotel on the river, having heard I was staying. He said he wanted to just shake my hand and gift me a River Moy half-marathon t-shirt; this was an event he was involved in. He then invited me, Tom and Aisling up to his restaurant, Crockets on the Quay. The random hospitality so far from home came with impeccable timing, exactly when I needed a lift. There were smiles all around again. As if the top-notch meal and dessert number 127 of the challenge wasn't enough, Alan even offered to join me for the next day's full marathon.

MARATHON 19: 14TH JUNE 2012

I must admit I was somewhat nervous about this marathon. I had struggled to walk to the previous day's finish line, never mind run to it, and the day before had been horrendous. Now I had this generous local joining me and expecting to run with me. There was an added pressure to deliver a run for him.

The magical hotel bed and bath candles worked a charm. Or maybe it was the filling three-course feast, the physio, or Alan's company on the run. I wasn't sure, and I didn't care why. I felt human again and was just happy to feel pain-free.

The conditions were bleak, with a deluge of rain pelting us side-on. The weather wouldn't drag me down on this one. Not even the Irish elements could dampen the wild scenery, running along rural Mayo's treelined roads, 'stone walls and the grass is green …', as The Saw Doctor's sang. We ran between and alongside Lough Conn and Lough Cullin, on through Cunnagher More

Bog Natural Heritage Area. *Now, that's what I'm talking about.*

Having the chats with my tour guide, I discovered Alan wanted to run an ultramarathon at some point in his future. Again, an ultramarathon is any distance beyond a marathon. He didn't think he was ready yet and wanted to do more training before breaking beyond the 42.2-kilometre mark. Little did he know, the stars would align much sooner than he'd planned. At kilometre 25.17, for the first time, I noticed my GPS watch wasn't moving beyond this number, despite our forward march.

'What's your Garmin reading there?'

'28.6, Al'.

'Shit on it anyway.'

With little choice, I stopped to click save to record the frozen 25.17-kilometre run. I had to reset my watch as if to start a new run. It was essential for me to do the run right by my standards, and that meant my watch having a record of 42.2 kilometres being covered on foot every day for the 35 days.

'0.1 kilometres left,' Alan informed me as we ran through Castlebar, looking at his watch which hadn't skipped a beat all day.

Having his watch going meant we could calculate what mine missed out on – 3.43 kilometres.

'I'm going to keep running until the two distances on my watch add up to the marathon distance. I know it will be over 45-kilometres in the end, but I don't want any doubts over my watch recordings.'

'I'll tag along so, an ultramarathon.'

'An ultramarathon. Today's your day.'

I got more satisfaction nudging Alan onto his longest ever run and his first ultra, than from the fact I'd completed marathon number 19.

The kindness towards the team and me, the picturesque scenery, reminding me of songs I'd heard and Alan's enjoyment and enthusiasm for running, made my time in Mayo unforgettable. The body held up for the entirety, even with the extra kilometres. 25.17 kilometres plus 17.03 kilometres, in a total marathon time of 5 hours and 31 minutes, ignoring the additional phantom 3.43 kilometres completed in the middle. *That will at least help make up for some of the wrong turns.*

Aisling was concerned about my dropping weight as she kept an eye on my Facebook posts, tracking the event's progress in images from day one. When she joined the team at the end of day 17, she had presented me with a cardboard tray of cartons containing high-calorie protein drinks. Ever the nurse, she instructed me to get at least one down me every day to stop me from wasting away to nothing. She'd thought I wasn't eating but witnessed it was quite the opposite. The weight I didn't have to lose was shredding off under the demands I was placing on my body and despite shovelling food away from dawn until dusk.

MARATHON 20: 15ᵀᴴ JUNE 2012

I was back on the mend, my body relatively pain-free, as I got moving south of Castlebar, towards Shrule. Sixteen kilometres in, I saw a Garda car pull over ahead of me. *They're going to give me a bollocking for running on this dangerous road, aren't they? They can shag off if they try remove me.* As I edged closer, the door opened. *Feck, it's definitely me they want to speak to.* I saw the peculiar sight of a pair of bare legs swinging out of the open passenger door in slow motion. I was greeted by James Carey, announcing himself as a local Garda who wanted to run with me for a bit. My nervous sweating turned immediately to laughter.

I later found Aisling and Tom had a similar experience. Sitting in the parked support car, they got a knock on their window, with the Garda looming over them.

'Are you with the man running these roads?' Immediately, Aisling thought I'd been run over.

'Shit. Oh no. Is he okay? We're his team.'

'I'm sure he's grand. We're just trying to track him down to join him.'

'You gave me a feckin' heart attack!' Aisling told him.

James ran with me for about 24 kilometres, and I learned of his plans to run five marathons in five consecutive days. As it turned out, we both had Gerry Duffy in our corner. James had tracked him down too, and Gerry had helped with a training plan.

It was a funny experience, hundreds of kilometres from home, running a marathon with a Garda, sharing tales and learning about our shared interests and challenges. The conversation was flying and it wiped past and future marathons from my mind as we ran effortlessly in chat, Garda James still in work mode, signalling traffic around us, much to my amusement.

'Welcome to Galway,' James announced as we stepped over the county border, just past Shrule.

I finished with the exact same time as the previous day, 5 hours and 31 minutes. No land speed record, of course, but

I was delighted to be running consistently and not to have the excruciating pains of the recent past.

After trekking cross country to help me out, Aisling's annual leave was up and she headed back to work in Waterford. It was all change. Tom's unpaid leave came to an end too. I was sad to see him go, Tom having smashed it out of the park in every aspect of his role over the 20 days. The only negative of having my childhood friend's undivided support for three weeks, was my obligation to buy him pints for the rest of his days. Well earned!

MARATHON 21: 16TH JUNE 2012

My brother, Evan, and his friend Declan Murphy stepped up to the plate on support team duties as we left Shrule and took aim at Headford.

I was on autopilot, with the only issue arising around the halfway mark. I was about three kilometres overdue a check-in with Ev and Declan for food, but they were nowhere to be found. If it were week one or two, I'd have been cursing them, but I'd become much less uptight about things not going exactly to plan. I was unrealistic at the start of the adventure. More seasoned now, I'd accepted there'd be punches and life was easier if I just rolled with them. There'd be wrong turns, injuries, malfunctioning watches, missed feeds but I had to get on with things the best I could and keep the positive vibes flowing. Things were hard enough without getting uptight over the minutiae.

Out of liquids and running on fumes once again, I was delighted to eventually find the men pulled in. The energy from the honking cars was great, but nothing quite prevents 'the wall' quite like snacks.

'Sorry Al, the road was too narrow and traffic too fast. We didn't feel safe pulling in anywhere sooner.'

'Don't sweat it. All good now, I'm fed and watered.'

With my Dublin and Belfast navigation experience amassed, we negotiated Galway City with ease. To be fair, it was all the lads. It helped big-time that Ev and Declan knew every pub in town from their student days, so we could orientate ourselves at all times!

Declan was in his late twenties and healthy but had had a recent health scare. He had a stent fitted in his heart – a small tube in the coronary artery, permanently helping to prop the artery open. He was mad to get involved and do some running but decided it was safer to take the less taxing option to cycle with me. The last thing we wanted fundraising for the Heart Foundation was any heart complications! Although, it might have seen a tenfold increase in donations with media lapping bad news up; nonetheless, we wanted Declan to remain safe and sound.

'You're not to overexert yourself.' God, I sounded like my mother.

'You're one to be talking,' Declan joked. It seemed I'd forever forfeited any right to be the voice of reason.

'Fair point.'

With Declan rolling beside me for six kilometres and Ev jogging with me for the last six kilometres, it was one of my better days for sure, kilometres ticking by without much strain. I finished in 5 hours and 19 minutes and jumped straight into the sea by Oranmore to cool off after a successful day.

MARATHON 22: 17TH JUNE 2012

Jogging away from Oranmore, my pasty skin was absorbing the morning's vitamin D through my thick layer of factor 50 sunscreen. With the cycling causing no ill effects, Declan insisted on running the first few kilometres. I didn't try to talk any sense into him on this occasion, knowing where I'd be told to go. He was happy, having his life recently threatened but now running free in the sun's glory. His joyous mood was infectious.

Once Declan left my side, things started to deteriorate, as my shaggin' knee was getting to me again. Things weren't looking too good, so I went back to the good aul' tried and tested strategy of running roughly a kilometre and walking for a tick for some sweet relief, without the expense of too much progress.

After kilometre eight, I returned to a consistent canter as the pain subsided. As with past experience, I learned not to dwell on how or why and just enjoyed the uninhibited running when I was afforded it. Today was like something out of a Tourism Ireland advertisement. The landscape had it all: dry stone walls, thatched cottages, mature large canopy trees, the ancient Dunguaire Castle, green expanses of fields with sheep and cattle, mountains and the sea. It was rural Ireland at its finest, with rare clear skies overhead. I was in my element, happy out.

Noting the sweat pouring off Ev and me as we passed through Ballyvaughan, Declan treated us to ice cream on the go. Our run's nutrition tactics garnered a few funny looks from the passing traffic. They acted like they'd never seen someone out for a jog while stuffing their face with ice cream!

Thankfully, the epic day didn't get spoiled by Corkscrew

Hill, with the finish line landing me at the foot of this godawful climb. *I'll worry about that tomorrow.*

Five hours and 42 minutes clocked. It was a tad slower, but not due to any injuries. I had allowed myself to take in the breath-taking scenery, not being too precious about the ticking clock.

MARATHON 23: 18ᵀᴴ JUNE 2012

The big bro and Declan were back to their day jobs after an enjoyable weekend of near pain-free progress.

The next dream team up was Joe Murphy and Stephen O'Rourke. Joe was a competitive swimmer who knew all about high-performance, having competed for senior national titles as a teenager. His competitiveness, attentive nature and team mentality, meant he was straight in to help with any and everything that might make my life a bit easier and give us the best chance of success. Steve was fresh off competing in Ireland's Strongest Man competition. Him lifting bags from the hotel out to the car was a sight to behold – like feathers they were: one bag, two bags, even five bags, like it was nobody's business! All in a day's work for big Steve.

I would have been screwed without my friends and family, who were consistently there for me throughout this journey. I was extremely fortunate to have competent, caring, enthusiastic and willing people give up their precious time to help a madman achieve a lofty ambition.

You'd think the chopping and changing of the team would make things complicated and bring teething issues. Not so. Everyone was switched on to their roles. They were all at the relaxed and humorous end of the scale too, which suited me down to the ground. Things were intense enough once the running started, and the light-hearted company was exactly what I wanted. The changing of the guard went smoothly each time and each change brought new enthusiasm and another friendly face to catch up and share the experience with. They all came to the challenge raring to go and injected a new lease of life into it.

I decided to be kind to my body and walked the infamous Corkscrew Hill, which welcomed me at the start of the day's proceedings. It was aptly named, climbing about 100 metres vertically within 1.5 kilometres, winding upwards, zigzagging back and forth on itself in consecutive hairpin turns. With that warmup mountain hike out of the way, I got jogging towards Lisdoonvarna and Doolin. I had been looking forward to this run since the start. Even though I was aware I'd have to work for the scenery, with the route's undulating terrain, I knew the effort would be even more worth it today. I'd finally get to see the Cliffs of Moher for the first time. On our road trip, Dad and I didn't have time for sightseeing. We were all business, trying to check as much of the route as possible in the limited time we had. My broken body had wrecked my plan to see the Giant's Causeway. I was in much better shape now and knew I'd have the time to take this beauty in.

Having Joe arrive for this marathon worked to our advantage. A keen surfer, he was familiar with the west coast spots and knew how to find the best vantage point, away from the throngs of tourists, where we could enjoy an epic view in peace. I paused my GPS watch at the halfway point, planning an extended break at the cliffs. We made our way down through a farmer's field and there they were, the mighty Cliffs of Moher. A sheer cliff-face was stretching as far as the eye could see, with the Atlantic Ocean resting at the feet of the awe-inspiring landmark. It was worth running 1,000 kilometres for the sight alone.

As we climbed up out of the field to get back to work, two stereotypical looking Irish farmers were standing at our exit point, flat caps, a big stick, wellies, V-neck jumpers and tweed jackets.

'We're going to be shot, lads.'

We cautiously approached with guilty heads, but Steve was quick off the mark to chat us out of trouble. The auld fellas were only too delighted to wish us all the best on our adventure and let our trespassing slide.

The second half of the marathon was all downhill, which made a nice change. Just so I couldn't enjoy the favourable terrain too much, the heavens decided to open and drown me. With the view from a height, I set my sights on the seaside surf town of Lahinch. DJ Joe hit the nail on the head as we rolled towards the town in the rain, choosing Ben Howard's upbeat tune, which became the anthem for the remainder of the tour:

'Keep your head up, keep your heart strong,

No, no, no, no,

Keep your mind set; keep your hair long.'

I threw the crew a smile and a shaka surfer's hand signal to indicate my approval – no more feckin' Bill Withers haunting me loudly on repeat! The town looked deceptively close, but I felt like I'd never get there, slowly winding my way down the meandering road, arriving some 90 minutes after first setting my sights on it. A little outside town, I crossed the day's finish line in a time of 5 hours and 28 minutes, which was becoming my steady average.

A woman named Susanne MacNamara, and her son, Reese, who was about eight, came to visit the hotel to wish us luck with the remainder of the journey. They gifted us a goodie bag of tasty treats to dig in to as well. In exchange, Reese wanted to race me outside the hotel. Needless to say, the speedy bugger won. Seeing the sheer enjoyment of his lit-up face during our short dash reminded me of myself at his age. After whooping me, his infectious smile and laughter were just priceless – a memorable end to yet another great day on the road.

MARATHON 24: 19TH JUNE 2012

I'd had a string of good days and today felt like it would be no different, the sun shining on my face. My times were becoming steadier, and I felt fewer ill effects on my body over the past couple of marathons.

Despite the run progressing and becoming less painful, the lack of donations was hanging over me like a dark cloud. Initially aiming to raise €35,000, there I was two-thirds of the way through, but the total was only around the €6,000 mark. It was demoralising, and I had to do something to tackle it.

Steve is heavily involved in the Irish music scene, so we thought we'd play to his strengths and put him on PR duty. On only his second day on the job, he secured a radio interview on the Colm Hayes Show, on 2FM. It wasn't my favourite pastime or my strong suit, but the running wasn't achieving enough donations on its own. I needed to be more bullish to promote the challenge if I was to raise anywhere near the original target figure.

A little after the stint on the radio, Joe shagged up and we missed a turn.

'I'm sorry, Al. Really sorry but we took a wrong turn. Sorry, dude.'

'It's grand. No worries. We'll just tip on ahead and find the next best route. Don't sweat it, Joe, honestly.'

He couldn't have been any more apologetic. I felt bad. His competitiveness meant he was hard on himself. I could have had a meltdown if this slip was on the east coast and my body was going from worse to worse, but I was relaxing more and more the further I made it. I was more confident than ever in being able to overcome anything. *What're another five kilometres in the scheme of things?* I now felt I could jog to the moon and back.

'Seriously, Joe, not a big deal. Not the first and won't be the last.'

He quickly found a solution, and we rolled onwards, finishing in a time of 5 hours and 27 minutes. It wasn't too shabby in light of stopping to do the plug on national radio.

MARATHON 25: 20TH JUNE 2012

I passed the first sign for home today, and it hit me hard. *Waterford.* I could not wipe the smile off my face and was getting tingling goosebumps all over. I felt elated. It's funny what does it for you. Completing a marathon was just routine, but a sign for Waterford – now that was something. When I looked at my watch, I clocked that my pace was nearly two minutes faster per kilometre than I usually go. It was reassuring the gears were still working, but I thought it best not the let the excitement get to me; best to hold off the sprint finish until I'm a bit closer than 420 kilometres from home.

Joe had lived in Limerick for a few years while studying and training out of the University of Limerick. He was on hand to navigate me through the city's twists and turns, as my dopey head floated on cloud nine, in a world of my own, reminiscing on the magnificent signpost. Making it out of the city, Joe threw on his runners to join me for a kilometre or two. Enjoying the experience, he stayed for 26 kilometres! *Not bad at all for a swimmer.* After my dire triathlon experience, I knew I'd barely last beside him for 10 metres in the water.

Down the main street in Adare, who do we see? Only my two former sprint training partners Thomas and Jessie Barr, and Thomas's girlfriend. A 'Run Forrest, run!' chant was going, as they waved their homemade banners saying 'Careful now!', 'Run Forrest, run!' and one with an image of the Success Kid meme and the words 'Ran my first marathon: didn't shit my pants.' It made my day. It didn't feel like a marathon this one, just time well spent with friends. Five hours and 19 minutes and feeling consistent once more.

With the number of wrong turns beginning to add up, we could now clearly see we were miles off the pre-prepared map targets. The concern remained about getting to the last day and being dumped with a mother of all runs to make up for past errors, completing all 35 marathons but being nowhere near home. Someone suggested starting the next marathon in the correct location, but I wasn't happy with leaving a gap. I decided to run an extra 10 minutes a day until we caught up with the 'X' on the expedition map. I didn't want to screw up my watch records, a beautiful tally of a 42.2-kilometre run, after a 42.2-kilometre run, so I chose to run the extra bits off the clock. I spun it as a relaxing cooldown. The guys saw it as me being cracked but respected that I wanted to cover every inch of the lap on my own steam. If I was running a lap of Ireland, I would do it properly, with integrity. Driving any distance to make up for errors, would compromise my vision and wasn't something I entertained even for a second.

MARATHON 26: 21ˢᵀ JUNE 2012

'I'm in bits, dude! My joints! I don't know how you're doing it,' said a worse for wear Joe. The verdict was in from the swimmer: running's hard.

My times were now consistently hovering at the 5 hours and 30 minutes mark. My body had hardened to the task at hand, and the adjustment was phenomenal. That's not to say it was a breeze by any stretch. Rainy and cold days still dragged and my body still ached immensely, particularly my knees and Achilles', although nothing like the acute pains suffered on the toughest of days along the Causeway Coast (Day 12) and through Sligo (Day 17).

Leaving Rathkeale, I climbed steadily out of Newcastlewest, through Abbeyfeale, out of County Limerick and into the Kingdom of Kerry. Only three counties left to go and the finish line was feeling more realistic with each passing kilometre. I had been looking forward to Kerry all along, hearing only great things but never having had a chance to see it for myself. With this section missed on the recce, I was in unchartered territory. Finishing the marathon just north of Castleisland, I stopped the watch at 5 hours and 30 minutes.

After four days on tour the two lads were 'bet'! I came out of my ice bath, not even 03:00 p.m., to find both of them snoring, fully clothed sprawled across their beds. I found it odd, slumber never came over me during the day; I was regimented in my 10:00 p.m. to 07:00 a.m. circadian rhythm but crashing into a siesta happened to every crew member after the morning in support. They had all earned the rest as far as I was concerned. Once Steve and Joe had booked food, physio and accommodation from the car, they were just left to feed and water me every five kilometres or so. It must have been like watching paint dry, my slowness hypnotising them to sleep by lunchtime.

With the day's running over and icing and feeding complete, I decided to visit the local doctor about the stinging sores that had been accumulating on my face since day 11. With years of intolerable acne, the pain of these sores was barely noticeable, but I'd never had them before and thought it best to get some medical advice since they were getting worse. The visit to the docs was hilarious. The GP didn't know what to make of me. In one sentence, wearing his doctor's hat, he'd tell me what I was doing was extreme and could cause a lot of harmful damage. The next sentence he'd switch to his runner's cap and exclaim how epic the whole concept was and how incredible it was that I had made it this far.

'The sores are a direct result of extreme stress. It's an

almighty strain you're putting on yourself, but they shouldn't be anything to worry about. I'd expect them to disappear with a few days complete rest after the finish. I'll give you a cream to help the process along.'

He gave me some anti-inflammatories to help with the joint pain too. Although used sparingly only on days that necessitated them, I had recently run out of my limited supply, with nine marathons left to run in as many days. I found they notably eased the grinding of my inflamed joints and tendons, and I wanted to hug the man for his medical support.

MARATHON 27: 22ND JUNE 2012

We experienced all four seasons during marathon 27, losing minutes to accommodate multiple gear changes to stay warm and dry. First, we made our way into Castleisland, via rural back roads, guarded by protective farm dogs. I'm not the best with guessing speed, but I'd say I ran a sub 10 second 100 metres to get away from the barking dog that gave chase. I was barely awake, and it was way too early in the morning for a sharp surge of adrenaline like that! My body hadn't moved that fast since I hung up my track spikes. It was a wonder my legs didn't fall off. Having bolted to safety, I folded over to catch my breath, my pulse racing.

In Farranfore, Mike Moriarty, the local Centra owner, was out to welcome my team and me to town, offering us deli delights and chocolates galore. You can't beat a bit of soundness to keep the spirits elevated. As we reached Killarney the sun broke through the dissipating clouds. The lush green mountains became visible and looked impressive in the town's background, although they made me somewhat concerned about my direction of travel. I hadn't paid a blind bit of notice to topography and elevations when mapping the route all those months ago. I now realised that might have been a mistake.

MARATHON 28: 23ᴿᴰ JUNE 2012

Once again, we had a changing of the guard. Joe headed back to Tramore to attend his weekend lifeguard shift, and Gavin Downey was in to replace him temporarily. Gavin was a member of Ferrybank AC too. He was an out and out distance runner, so we had never run together. Given Gav's background, it was no surprise he laced up straight away to accompany me into the vastness of the Kerry mountains. I was surprised to hear he wanted to go the full distance and complete his first-ever marathon with me. Boy, did Gav pick one!

Mountain inclines, wind, spectacular views and rain sums up the day's marathon: most of the things that spring to mind when you think of Kerry. I loved seeing my country on foot, taking it all in at a steady pace. This landscape was certainly contending for the top spot, and I was glad to be out amidst it all, despite the difficulty.

Those that know the Ring of Kerry, know it's difficult in a car, it's torturous on a bicycle and you'd be daft to run the steep, narrow winding roads. The gradient was relentless as we looped upwards around dodgy blind bends. The course seemed to be the place to be for cyclists, testing their legs up the famous Moll's Gap and on to Ladies View. We didn't want to be splattered on the windshield of a tourist bus or flattened by the packs of riders coming head-on, freewheeling downhill, swooping around the corners. We often opted to zig-zag from one side of the road to the other, for safety.

The cyclists seemed amused seeing two runners along the route so far from town.

'Are you lost?' they'd quip, whizzing downhill or huffing and puffing their way uphill past us.

'Where the feck are you off to, lads?'

'Waterford!'

Our synchronized response turned a few puzzled heads as they did some quick maths and geography.

My eyes didn't want the panoramic postcard scenery to stop, but the legs screamed, 'When does this road go downhill?' It was a laugh or cry kind of section, as we climbed and climbed and climbed. Every time we thought we had reached the top as it levelled off, we would turn a corner and have another hill taunting us. We chose to roll up our sleeves and laugh at the test.

My parents were back on tour. They pulled in ahead of us, having driven three hours to see me. I hadn't seen them since my dad left to represent the FAI at the European Football Championships in Poland, way back in Belfast on marathon 10. Unfortunately for Ireland, we were dismal in the football tournament, but the early knockout meant Dad could be home to spend more time on the challenge.

'Quite a route you picked, Al,' he winked.

Out in the elements, on the back-breaking course with my friends and now my family with me, it was a dream turned into a reality.

Gav would have loved a three-hour first marathon, and was probably well capable too, but he held back at my granny pace. I was chuffed with our 5 hours and 39 minutes in the context of how far I had come and the vertical climbing involved in the day's testing mountainous route. Although not a racer's marathon, Gavin was grinning ear to ear after the adventurous day.

'When else would you run a marathon up a mountain?'

Unfortunately for me, the local physio only had a slot available at 09:00 p.m. I had to make a tough choice. Food was a priority since I was still whittling away, despite gorging every day. Sleep was vital too; I was out for the count as soon as my head hit the pillow, sleeping like a baby and waking fresh as a daisy. I didn't want to mess up my finely tuned body clock. On balance, I had to turn down the body mechanic for the first time. My body might regret it, but I was in good nick all things considered. I felt it was better for my general wellbeing to catch-up and enjoy quality family time, with a big feed, in front of some live trad music – the perfect end to a challenging but memorable and rewarding day.

NINE

THE LONG HOME STRAIGHT

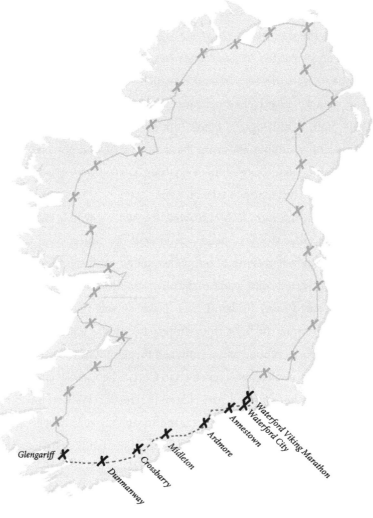

DAY 29 – DAY 35:

Glengariff–Dunmanway–Crossbarry–Midleton–Ardmore–
Annestown–Waterford City–Waterford Viking Marathon

MARATHON 29: 24TH JUNE 2012

Picking up where we had finished the previous day, I had a right aul' climb to kick things off. Steve, Gavin and I were high in Kerry's mountains, just shy of the County Cork border. It was hard work to start the day, but there was a sight to behold at the top. The team and I paused to smell the roses, taking in the vast expanse of the valley and peaks behind us which stretched to the horizon; the road I had travelled appeared as a pencil-thin line from up this high. Admiring the land's immensity, I felt proud standing at the top, thinking about the hard work that had got me to the viewpoint. I had conquered everything Kerry threw at me; I was sad to leave but ready to take on Cork.

Turning our backs on what we had achieved, facing the challenge that still lay ahead, we entered the tiniest road tunnel I'd ever seen. It was just about wide enough to fit the support car, a low untreated ceiling and rocks all around looking like they had been hacked away by hand. The darkness was illuminated only by the glimmer of light from either end of the black hole. Our playful shouts echoed as we frolicked through. On the other side, a road sign officially welcomed us to Cork. The views were no less impressive than on the Kerry side of the border. We were heading down from the high ground, taking in the surrounding emerald hills, a blanket of dense woodlands and farmlands delineated by dry stone walls, the sea in view in the distance.

'Unreal, lads, isn't it?'

'Pretty feckin' nice alright!'

I was in a state of perfect contentment, running into the unknown with my friends and seeing parts of my spectacular country for the first time, seeing a bit more money donated for the causes each day.

Whilst entering undiscovered lands had many positives, there were downsides too. We didn't know what lay ahead and there was no time for informed re-routing, so we'd just have to go for it. The support car was driving back towards me. Something was up.

'We have an ... *interesting* section ahead, Al. There's a sign with a hiker on it, and you have to open a gate to get through. We've double-checked and think that's where your map is sending us.'

This could hardly be right? I thought.

'Are you sure?'

We pulled out the maps and conferred with our phones. The N71 swooped, wisely, in a big arch around the hill and through the Glengarriff Woods Nature Reserve. My route shot straight as the crow flies up a boreen and into the sticks.

'Want to follow the road around or see where this trail leads?'

'Fuck it, let's follow the planned route.'

We were proper off-roading, going where Google Street View couldn't fit, two dirt tyre tracks with grass running up the middle. Adding to the remote path's mystique were abandoned cars, bathtubs, tractors and even a boat. Suboptimal running conditions, you might say, but a peculiar and funny experience with Steve hauling the bicycle nonetheless and we made it through.

My parents found us when we got back on the tarmac and I convinced Mam to join me for a while, despite her initial reluctance.

'No, no, I'll just be slowing you down.'

'It's not run at all costs, Mam. The company would be nice for a while, c'mon will ye, and stretch your legs?' Off we went up the road together, following the roadside posts with hiker symbols, indicating what kind of route this was.

My mam had had a real tough year, being a pillar of strength and caring for Dad. I didn't help matters, with her fears about my run adding to her stress levels. From my perspective, there were a lot worse things than charity ultra-running to get entangled in, so I didn't feel too guilty for creating the extra burden. She was a lot more at ease now by day 29, thank God. She was more relaxed having seen me still smiling and enjoying myself this far into the challenge, importantly, having avoided any hospital trips. Sharing steps with my mam and having her there despite her fears and initial reluctance meant the world. Her simply being there was all I needed and to have Dad drive along with us meant I couldn't ask for more. I was a lucky man.

After hugging my mother for tagging along for a short walk, it was time to get running again. After another few kilometres, things were hotting up.

'Want an ice cream, Al?' my dad shouted from the car.

'Yeah, g'wan sure. Thanks, a mil.' We stopped in Ballylickey, a seaside village north of Bantry, to devour some sweet cold sugar together. It cooled my head and warmed my heart to share the simple moment with Dad. This marathon had it all.

Refreshed, we moved south, the unresearched route greeting us with another peculiarity. *Not again!* Another line plotted on the map was leading me up a laneway with grass up the middle of it; this off-road lane was as narrow as the first, but even steeper. This marathon was turning into more of an orienteering adventure, than a road run. *I guess you have to be careful what you wish for, don't you?* Kerry and West Cork were ticking all the adventure boxes I wanted at the start of my dream, but they were also ensuring no let-up in days of hard graft.

Six hours and 20 minutes: my third slowest, only behind the torturous days along the north coast and through Sligo. It was a world apart from those days, however. I was slow because of steep off-road sections forcing me to decelerate to a walk and because I took the time to enjoy my family's company, not because I was falling apart like in the days gone by. I felt strong and was as happy as Larry to have taken a big turn, now officially heading east on the long home straight to Waterford.

MARATHON 30: 25ᵀᴴ JUNE 2012

The conditions were sweet: no rain, warm, with clouds blocking direct sunlight on my pale skin – a prime environment for a sweaty, pasty white boy.

It was my first day with just a one-person support team; Steve was still by my side. The route was a straight shot from Dunmanway, through Bandon and into Crossbarry. Out of the mountains and back to level pavement, I was counting my lucky stars. As picture-perfect as the last few days had been, they had been a hard slog. Having been restrained on the inclines, it felt nice to take the chains off and stretch my legs again. My confidence was sky-high, having 29 marathons down and only half a dozen left, with the mountainous section behind me. I wasn't home and dry just yet, with over 250 kilometres to go, but I was relatively close and relaxed my self-preservation policy slightly.

With my parents gone home and Steve busy finding food and accommodation, there was no procrastination, just freedom to run.

I only stopped briefly at the support vehicle twice, quick pitstops to refuel.

'Feeling good, Steve. Gotta run. Let me know of any issues. Thanks.'

'I have everything looked after. You're moving today. Keep it up,' Steve shouted as I legged it off.

I ended up clocking my second fastest marathon of the challenge – 4 hours and 59 minutes. It was only slightly slower than marathon number one. I was delighted with my achievement but more delighted with just how good it felt not to have excruciating pain or vertical gradients forcing me to take walking breaks.

'There's still five to go, man. Maybe hold off on any sprint finish?'

Steve was dead right. Five-and-a-half hours seemed to be my sweet spot. It was fast enough to allow plenty of recovery time, not protracting the time on my feet too much, while slow enough not to inflict much damage. There was no need to be shaving 30 minutes off. I needed to stay restrained and disciplined.

MARATHON 31: 26TH JUNE 2012

Joe was back for more punishment, helping Steve guide me through Cork City. Having dropped my mam home, Dad was back again, as supportive as ever.

The N71 was a bit of an uphill struggle coming into the city from Crossbarry, but I've learnt along the way that what goes up must come down. Unfortunately, in my experience to this point, I also knew what goes down goes back up, sooner than I'd like. I got suspicious when I reached sea level. *Shite, there's going to be a hill soon, isn't there?* As predicted, after making my way across the River Lee at the end of Cork City's main street, my team point me up Summerhill. *Feck sake, ugh.*

I was melting from the heat and uphill exertions, changing my sweat-drenched t-shirt multiple times to try to stay comfortable. Reaching the point of the marathon where decency fades, I chucked my top into the wash bag and ran bare-chested. I should have known better with my snow-white skin! The sun cruelly imprinted a glowing stencil of the hydration pack on my back. I was a running tribute to the Cork flag, paying homage to the red and white of the Rebel County I was passing through.

With more stops, hills and the high temperature, I accepted a slower time of 6 hours and 2 minutes. The time felt irrelevant. All I could think of was crossing into the Déise – my home county – on the next marathon.

MARATHON 32: 27TH JUNE 2012

I had just got moving from Midleton when I spotted a train crossing coming up in the distance. Edging closer, the lights started flashing, and the warning alarm sounded. I made a burst for it, not wanting progress halted just as I was getting going. Too slow. I was half tempted to see if I still had my hurdles technique but thought better of it as I calculated my stride pattern. My football coach was right. All this distance work would zap my speed. Losing the sprint, I just had to stand there dejected, waiting with the frustrated commuters who were forming a traffic jam.

I had to stop two more times for radio interviews, on Newstalk and Beat 102-103, media now taking more interest, with Steve's persistence on the promotional side of things and with the likelihood of completing the challenge increasing. The chore detracted from the running experience, but the donation tally was still disappointing – only around €7,000. I didn't feel it even came close to matching the effort I'd made, running 32 consecutive marathons. Assured in my ability to make the finish line, I needed to divert more time and energy to promotional work, to make the whole endeavour more worthwhile. I couldn't argue with the results, the listeners and readers injecting donations after each piece.

Interviews out of the way and returning to running, my back began stinging strangely. It wasn't an internal back injury like my day in Dublin, but more of a surface wound. It didn't feel like sunburn either. I ignored it the best I could for as long as I could until the sensation could be ignored no more.

'Is my back okay, lads?' I inquired, lifting my t-shirt up for Joe and Steve to inspect the situation.

'No. No, it is not. You've got foam all over you and a big red rash. The good news is that you don't have a white patch from yesterday's sunburn anymore. The red rash has filled that milk bottle rectangle in nicely.'

The hydration pack had rubbed off on washing up capsules

in the boot of the car. Once strapped to my back, the warmth, sweat, and friction caused a washing machine reaction, frothing the detergent up and setting my skin ablaze. *That's life, huh?* Just when I thought I'd covered all the bases and seen it all, a rogue thorn reminded me that comfort and stability are never constants.

While cursing my misfortune, I got a welcome surprise and distraction. My former football team captain, Paul Farrelly, ventured out to run with me for a kilometre. Again, a gesture of thoughtfulness to ease the day's sting just when I needed it most.

Finally, the moment arrived when I breached the border back into my home county. What a feeling! I was so happy I leapt up in pure delight and hugged the pole, supporting the words: Contae Phort Láirge COUNTY WATERFORD.

Fog rolled in as we continued deeper into the home territory, but I soon crossed the finish line as the hazy hazard engulfed us, the opposite side of the road now impossible to see. After quickly spraying the marker, we retreated from the roadside and out of harm's way. Checking my watch, it read 5 hours and 59 minutes.

My own people were spoiling me. Ardmore's five-star Cliff House Hotel offered to accommodate us for a night.

'We only have a suite available, if that's okay, sir?'

'Sure, if it has a bed, I'm more than happy,' not knowing the difference between a suite and a non-suite.

We were escorted to our room like noblemen, although looking like dirtbags. The elegant hotel porter opened the door for us to look inside.

'I hope this is suitable and you enjoy your stay.'

We lost our shit when he closed the door. There were stairs

and a second storey in the hotel room!

'Is this okay!? *Only* a suite left, they said!?'

We would live like kings for the rest of the day. We cannonballed into the sea off the pier wall, the breath-taking immersion like a defibrillator shocking my system back to life. Refreshed, just the right side of hypothermic, it was back to the swanky mansion of a suite for treatment from Aisling Hayden, the day's physio, offering the first house call of the challenge. For the evening, we indulged in a fine feast put on for us by the local White Horses Restaurant. Oh, it was never nicer to be on home turf and floating on top of the world. Spoiled rotten, I was!

MARATHON 33: 28TH JUNE 2012

For the first time, we couldn't find the start line. We had always sprayed bright canary yellow paint on the roadside at the end of each day with the completed marathon's number. We'd take photographs of the immediate surroundings and screengrab our location on Google Maps. It was no use today, though, with number 32 nowhere to be found. Yesterday's blanket of fog made the orientating finish photos redundant, and we'd forgotten to screengrab the location in our hurry out of harm's way and off the road. The only option I had was to drive back towards Youghal until we came to a landmark, I was 110% sure I had run past. I knew I was adding a few kilometres to the overall distance by doing this. I much preferred the peace of mind from running further than planned to finding out later that I'd taken a shortcut by starting ahead of the previous day's finish line. Nobody would care, and it wasn't any official record attempt with adjudicators, but I needed to satisfy myself. The lads thought I was mad backtracking so far.

'Ah here lad, we definitely passed this point yesterday, surely?'

'I think so. I'm not 100%. Let's keep going back to be safe.'

Once satisfied, I got running. Yesterday's fog was still lingering, making for dangerous conditions in the hard shoulder of the lorry thoroughfare into Dungarvan. The hi-vis bib was implemented, with Steve joining on the bicycle to increase our visibility and safety.

My dad was on the road cheering me on again, bringing his old friends Bill and Lillian along for extra encouragement on my homeward leg. I had conquered the mountain summit and was nearly back to base camp with local support building.

I ran along the Copper Coast European Geopark, with a pep in my step, taking in the fresh sea breeze and sights not too dissimilar to the remarkable Causeway Coastline. I was mad at myself for not previously taking the time to fully appreciate the wild coastal route that was right on my doorstep.

'Were these views and this road always here, lads?'

For the last time, I got to spray down the marker to indicate the end of marathon 33 and the start of marathon 34. There would be no need for a spray-painted finish line after number 34, as day 35 would see me joining the hundreds of participants running the Waterford Viking Marathon.

MARATHON 34: 29TH JUNE 2012

Having patched me up all year, Siobhan Fitzpatrick, was out to join me for the first 13 kilometres of the penultimate marathon.

She had to hang on for a while, as did I, twiddling our thumbs itching to go, but having to wait for the RTÉ Radio 1 producer to patch me through to answer their questions, live. Distracted, I muddled my way through the interview and jumped out of the support car.

'Will we run a lap of Ireland so?' I asked Dad, Ev and Siobhan.

'We're here now, might as well.'

A few kilometres in, I passed my old football club in Tramore, where John Power and Paul Power had assembled a welcoming committee. You couldn't beat the home support! In a world increasingly full of begrudgers and trolls cutting the backs off everyone, I seemed to be surrounded by people that wanted only the best for me and shared in the joy of winning with me.

Siobhan misjudged the distance from the start line to where she'd parked her car along the route. I could only laugh when this realisation dawned as we ticked over 13 kilometres, knowing the car was still an age away.

Dad and Ev pulled up alongside in the support car to check on us.

'Siobhan only planned to do 13 kilometres, but her car is about eight kilometres ahead,' I explained, knowing this route quite well from training.

'We can give you a spin?' my dad offered.

'God, no. You're grand Milo. I haven't the training done, but I'll manage. He's after running around the country. You can't be driving me to my feckin' car.'

I knew she was concerned about nearly doubling the

distance, but to Siobhan's credit, she recalibrated and told the question marks in her head to feck off. She wanted to keep going, refusing to raise the white flag many would have opted for.

I'd witnessed Alex Flynn, and Gavin Downey both run their first marathons with me. I enjoyed accompanying Seán Drohan on his first half-marathon and Tom Davies, his first three-kilometre road run. Sean Kinsella took the biscuit with completing his first, second *and* third marathon, and Alan Murphy did his first ultramarathon. Now, Siobhan was going beyond the limit she'd set herself earlier in the day. It was all mighty stuff: highly motivating and rewarding to be partly responsible for everyone breaking their previous limits. I loved just being there, sharing those experiences with them and seeing the glow of satisfaction on their faces after giving that bit more. The positivity had a way of rubbing off on those around them and always boosted my spirits, inspiring me to keep going.

With Siobhan sore but safely to her car, I continued out the back roads from Tramore to Dunmore, twisting and turning through the open countryside while trying to avoid the pothole booby traps. I spotted my father driving back towards me. I knew by now that the car coming back was only a bad thing. I wasn't wrong.

'Some bad news, Al, RTÉ are ahead.'

I knew the national TV station were out filming a piece for the six o'clock news. I crossed my toes, fingers, and eyes hoping it would do some good for the final tally we were still well short of. By now, we knew the importance of the publicity, so I knew their presence wasn't the bad news Dad was talking about.

'They've plopped themselves at the top of the hill out of Ballymacaw. Think you'll manage a quick sprint up it?'

'Ah, for feck sake. Out of all the places they could shoot me running. I'll give it a lash.'

'Good man, Al.'

They'd only gone and picked the steepest bit of road of the entire day's route. I took a 30-second breather behind a bush when out of view of the cameramen, storing up enough energy to make a go at the hill. If I was just sauntering past at my typical pace, I'd have no chance of connecting with and inspiring viewers to dig into their pockets. I'd need to floor it – well, by 35 consecutive marathon standards anyway.

The sun was glistening off the sea as I made it into the beautiful village of Dunmore East, welcomed by heckling seagulls chasing the trawlers into the harbour. With Mam hard at work in the hospital, it was a boy's day out. Dad and I sat on the wall overlooking the sandy beach, while Ev laced up his runners to join me for the last 15 kilometres.

'Didn't think we'd be here after you showing me the Eddie Izzard documentary, did you?'

'Not at all,' he laughed.

'Me neither,' I said with a big smile. 'You're a bad influence.'

It was a perfect stretch into the city, talking with Ev about the highs and lows of the adventure and how unbelievable it was having Dad driving along with us after his arduous recovery ordeal. I was dreaming with my eyes open.

We made it to the finish line in the People's Park in a time of 5 hours and 37 minutes. A small group of family and friends were there to share in the celebrations as I joined up the last dots, back to where I had started five weeks earlier.

'I told you I'd do it, didn't I?' I joked with my parents.

The pints would have to wait, though, as I needed to register myself for the Viking Marathon. The race organisers presented me with pins and my race number, number 35. I headed home to recuperate and follow my recovery routine as usual, with dopamine flooding my system and feeling the buzz of the moment. Not a hope. I wasn't 10 seconds in the door before being handed a basket of washing that needed hanging on the line. I may have just become the first person to run a lap of Ireland, but my family were going to ensure my feet remained firmly on the ground.

MARATHON 35: 30TH JUNE 2012

The finale had arrived. I did my usual morning routine: up at 07:00 a.m., stretch and foam roll, two bowls of plain porridge and out the gap. I made my way onto The Mall, in Waterford City for the beginning of the end.

As with day one of the marathon journey, the butterflies returned, entering the crowded street of runners. There was a lot more hullabaloo than I was used to on the beautifully solitary open road: people asking questions, shaking my hand and wanting photos and such. It was nice to be appreciated, but I was glad I didn't follow Dean, Gerry and Ken's blueprint all the same. I was accustomed to and fell in love with the peace of solo running and found the hanging about at the frantic start zone a bit alien.

I later discovered the race organisers had been looking for

me to start with my toe to the tape, right up the front, but nobody informed me. Just as well, since I would have been a hazard getting in the way of the speedsters. I was content hiding on my own near the middle of the herd, the charity, unsurprisingly, having secured zero 'run with Alan' participants, none I was told of anyway.

The gun blasted at 09:00 a.m. I felt like the entire field passed me during the first kilometre, along the city's riverfront. I could have been dead last for all I cared. I was happier than a seagull with a stolen chip. This day was all about soaking up the atmosphere and taking as much pleasure from the freedom and good health I was afforded to participate.

Randomers encouraged me, patting me on the back as they flew past me. The last thing I wanted to do was get cocky and head off at a gallop, only to blow up. I started reserved, not wanting to risk missing the pub in the evening, for the sake of marathon personal record. There was just no need. I was tempted for a while but had to remind myself of Gerry's advice once more. The goal was 35 marathons in 35 consecutive days, not 34 marathons and see how fast I could run the 35th. *Imagine keeling over now? Nice and slow. Don't be a twat.*

I was tranquil running the secluded backroads at a sensible pace to Tramore, which would be the halfway point. Through the countryside, away from the crowds, I reflected on the journey – how bonkers it all was. With only four weeks of training and one long run to my name, I had foolishly stood on the Dublin City Marathon start line on the 31st October 2011, as probably the most inexperienced distance runner in the field. Fast forward only eight months, now I had close to 50 marathons to my name, probably making me one of the most experienced marathoners in the field. Dad, a stroke victim in March 2011, immobile and without speech; dragging himself up the steps in Wembley in May 2011; back driving in June 2011; now back working with the FAI at the Euros and supporting me around Ireland in the summer of 2012. What a whirlwind journey for us both.

The well-wishers who congregated in Tramore snapped me out of my daydream. They lined the streets and were egging all the participants on. Unconsciously, I accelerated. It's difficult not to increase speed and effort with all the energy the hollering onlookers were channelling towards the road runners. I found a quicker pace comfortable and liked how it felt.

Ev was on his bicycle, checking in on his partner, Deirdre, and me.

'How you feeling, Al?'

'Good as new! Where's Dee? How's she getting on?'

'She's a bit ahead. Maybe a kilometre. Struggling, though.'

'I'll go say "hi".'

We chatted and laughed as I wound the pace up a notch or two. I was loving this one, picking off the runners who whizzed past me at the start, visibly paying the price for their early enthusiasm. *Oh, been there, buddy*, I thought.

'Free' was the word on my mind. At this point I hadn't a care in the world and felt indestructible, like I could run forever. It was incredibly liberating to stretch my legs at a quicker pace, knowing there was only half a marathon to go, with little to no risk of failure left. All my upcoming diary consisted of was nursing a hangover the next day, and there was nothing planned beyond tomorrow.

Everything over the last year had been working towards getting my degree and getting to this finish line. I was going to make the most of the day and worry about the future later.

I slowed when I caught up with Deirdre to see if she was enjoying it. Stupid question. Like a lot on this inaugural marathon, it was her first. She was battling. I thought it best I took my excessive energy levels elsewhere, instead of annoying her with my peppiness. When I was going through hell on some of my marathons, the last thing I'd want is some cheery fucker rubbing in how glorious the day was going.

'You're doing great; keep it up, Dee. I'll leave you to it and see you at the finish.'

'Ugh, g'wan.'

My old kitchen colleague, Stephen Mullally, joined along on his bicycle too, forming a little posse.

'Either of you see that old-age pensioner they announced at the start? She's on her 107th marathon apparently.'

'Think she's ahead.'

'Ah here, I'm not having that,' I smiled.

I was floating, shifting up through the gears and gliding past the other participants when I spotted the machine in her late seventies on the other side of the road, which looped back on itself. There were only about four kilometres to go.

'Oh, I have her now, lads.'

Yes, I was racing down possibly the oldest person in the field and may have been taking great enjoyment out of passing the lady, but that veteran competitor wouldn't have had it any other way, I'm sure of it! After just about passing out the admirable Ms

Kay O'Regan, I sailed through the last kilometres into the Regional Sports Centre. The track which hosted the marathon's finish line was my old stomping ground. Where better to finish than where my running days had started way back in primary school, the place where I'd spent thousands of hours making friends, falling in love and honing my health and resilience?

I somersaulted my way across the line in celebration, clocking a time of 4 hours and 35 minutes; my fastest marathon of the 35-day adventure. I could have died a happy man at this moment, feeling I'd lived a full life despite my youth. It was an emotional finish, seeing my proud father, with his sister, Cora, brother, Liam, my mam and Ev, all there to share in the family success. We knew how different everything could have gone for Dad, for me, for us.

Dad and I stood together for a photo under the finish line banner. It was a finish line for me, of course, but I felt it was a symbolic finish line of sorts for Dad too, given his inspirational transformation back near to his former self. We did alright for ourselves, rebounding back, making the best of a bad situation and turning our tragedy into triumph. Yesterday's sacrifices had paid off and we earned our moment of joy and contentedness.

TEN:

COOL DOWN AND REFLECTIONS

MUCH DONE, MORE TO DO

I left plenty in the tank to hit the pub and club after the Viking Marathon, and of course the obligatory 03:00 a.m. burger and chips afterwards too. Better yet, I didn't have to pay for a single pint all night. *I should do this more often.* The vibe in town was electric. Everyone was out blowing off some steam after completing their challenging training schedule and passing the final exam on the tarmac.

It was a strange feeling the next day, with no alarm set and with nowhere to run. My mind was saying, *water, two plain bowls of porridge and stretch,* but my mam had the full works cooked up: rashers, eggs, sausages, pudding, blahs and a pot of tea to wash down all the good stuff.

I had crossed the 35-marathon finish line, and I wanted to relax, but calls were coming in thick and fast from the media. I had been long fed up with the promotional aspect but knew the difference each little article or minute of airtime was making to the fundraising total. The post-run week of shite-talking did the trick. It was a productive week's work with the total more than doubling to €15,317. I was glad I hadn't quit before completing the 35 – the donations hinged on media exposure, and the media exposure hinged on me finishing the run. Failing to complete the run or do the media work would have left me at around €7,000. The late surge was a relief and added to the sense of achievement, knowing all I went through was not in vain, with a respectable sum of money to donate. It was miles from my original fundraising target, and lower than similar challenges but, feeling I had left no stone unturned, I could hold my head high for trying my best to contribute. My dad and I proudly presented €10,117 to the Irish Heart Foundation, €2,600 to the brain injury unit at the NRH and €2,600 to the Football Village of Hope. It wasn't too shabby for a years' work. Not too shabby at all.

EPILOGUE

All good things must come to an end. Life levelled out from the exhilarating peaks and miserable troughs between the point of Dad's stroke and presenting our cheques to the charities.

Life just went on. With no Town Planning work in recessionary Ireland to put my undergraduate degree to use, I pursued a postgraduate course in Cardiff, Wales. At the same time, Dad resumed his full duties with the Football Association, as Chairman of the International Committee.

Dad had been very lucky, but luck alone did not lead to his astonishing recovery. It was all heart and hard work to ensure a spectacular return. He wasn't in perfect health after the traumatic stroke experience. Still, he had the quality of life he wanted and could enjoy time with his family, holidays to the sun in Portugal, walks on Tramore and Woodstown beaches, football and hurling matches and tea and biscuits with friends. That's what he fought hard for – a return of independence and freedom. He rose, only to fall time and time again, cursing the rehabilitation process's difficulty. He did not relent. Doing a little bit of work every day, he was back to 95%, savouring life's simple pleasures once more, with a newfound appreciation for how quickly it might be stolen.

Between quitting athletics, which I'd devoted half my life to, experiencing a messy end to a long-term relationship and then coming within a hair's breadth of my dad dying – it was a hell of a lot for a young college boy to process all at once. With nothing to lose by trying, I managed to get creative and reorientate myself, working towards an engaging and worthwhile pursuit. Coming up with a plan and, more importantly, implementing it, gave me back a feeling of control. Life wasn't just happening to me: I was imagining with my able mind, I was moving with my able body and I was contributing with my able heart, grateful for all three. I was alive, healthy and operating in the knowledge that life is short.

For all the ordeals that came from my decision to go on the offensive and pursue my dream, it was time well spent rambling those mucky training trails and learning as I went. As for the challenge itself, I never felt more alive than in those 35 days. It was life wedged into five weeks. Bad days of pain and misery seemed like they would never end, and things could only get worse with such a long road ahead. Good days were euphoric, thinking life doesn't get much better than this. Both ends of the spectrum passed eventually, which taught me that hard times would pass and so too would the good times. It's all temporary. In the hard times, positive steps, even just an inch a day, will eventually break through the difficulty and the feeling will be replaced. In the good times, hard times lie ahead for sure. Make hay while the sun shines. Try to ignore the distractions and focus on the things of most value: your physical and mental health, your time, your family and friends, your passions. Immerse yourself in nature and smell those roses while you're fortunate enough to have the pleasure.

Thank you for reading my 'Marathon Man' story. I hope you enjoyed joining me on my journey and would love to see your Amazon reviews to help me towards my next book, where I swim the length of Ireland – 500 kilometres of sea swimming.

ACKNOWLEDGEMENTS

First and foremost, a huge thank you to the medical staff of the Waterford University Hospital, St Patrick's Hospital, Waterford, and the National Rehabilitation Hospital, Dún Laoghaire, for all the care and attention you gave my dad.

Thank you to everyone who made an effort to donate to my chosen charities and furthered their missions. Thanks to those who left a 'like', a message of encouragement, or shared the event online. The kindness cost nothing but did not go unnoticed, helping lift the team's mood, spread awareness and ultimately increase the charitable donations.

I am eternally indebted to my friends and marathon support crew, Gavin Downey, Seán Drohan, Aisling Kennedy, Sean Kinsella, Declan Murphy, Joe Murphy and Stephen O'Rourke. You guys made the journey what it was – a trip of a lifetime.

In a group of stars, I have to single out one for special attention, Tom Davies. Without a notion or care for running, you still took three weeks out of your career and life to help me achieve my dream. Your companionship to make me smile and your professionalism in salvaging the near-empty spreadsheet, while getting me to where I needed to be each day, enabled me to do what I did. I cannot thank you enough for your support, old buddy.

A large chunk of the charitable donation was generated off the back of associated fundraising events. Thank you to all those volunteers who gave up their time and made an effort to get the donation tally off the ground.

Gerry Duffy and Gerry Deegan: your training guides for this beast were essential to its success. I would have been lost without your kind assistance. Thank you for going out of your way to share your time, knowledge and expertise.

Siobhan Fitzpatrick, Roy Brennan and Rory Carthy, thank you for beating your pointed thumbs, elbows and needles into my battered muscles throughout my training period. Thank you also to all the physios, physical therapists and masseuses that provided me respite along the unforgiving road. Even the prospect of reaching your care was enough to ease the struggle on hard days.

A sincere thank you is owed to my event clothing sponsors, 53 Degrees North and Alfie Hale Sports; event car sponsor, John Flood's Dungarvan Nissan Garage, and every hotel, bar, and restaurant that fuelled the journey.

My flatmate for the year of the marathon, Simon Cody, your humour, friendship and support eased the burden of a loaded couple of months. I can't forget a massive word of praise and thanks for all the professional graphic design work too – the fashion show posters, the car branding and this entire book! You're my boy, Blue.

Thanks, Darren Doheny, for the slick photography which made me at least look like I knew what I was up to.

My athletics coaches, Brid and Alan Golden, Jim and Andy Kidd, John Shields, and Tramore AFC coaches, Paul Power, Paul O'Neill and Tommy Griffin: your love of, and commitment to, sports were an inspiration growing up. I think I can speak for all the footballers and runners that you've guided over the years, in saying a big thank you all for giving the time and attention to teaching us, keeping us out of trouble and on a healthy productive path.

Finally, my partner, Karolina: thank you with all my heart for the love and encouragement during the writing of this book, for the proofreading and for not killing me for continually waking you up to type before going to my day job.

APPENDIX 1 - MARATHON TIMES

Day 1 – 4hrs 51m

Day 2 – 5hrs 12m

Day 3 – 5hrs 20m

Day 4 – 5hrs 38m

Day 5 – 6hrs 04m

Day 6 – 5hrs 48m

Day 7 – 5hrs 25m

Day 8 – 5hrs 56m

Day 9 – 5hrs 04m

Day 10 – 5hrs 35m

Day 11 – 5hrs 47m

Day 12 – 6hrs 34m

Day 13 – 6hrs 09m

Day 14 – 5hrs 56m

Day 15 – 5hrs 44m

Day 16 – 5hrs 37m

Day 17 – 6hrs 25m

Day 18 – 5hrs 58m

Day 19 – 5hrs 31m

Day 20 – 5hrs 31m

Day 21 – 5hrs 19m

Day 22 – 5hrs 42m

Day 23 – 5hrs 28m

Day 24 – 5hrs 27m

Day 25 – 5hrs 19m

Day 26 – 5hrs 30m

Day 27 – 5hrs 49m

Day 28 – 5hrs 39m

Day 29 – 6hrs 20m

Day 30 – 4hrs 59m

Day 31 – 6hrs 02m

Day 32 – 5hrs 59m

Day 33 – 5hrs 54m

Day 34 – 5hrs 37m

Day 35 – 4hrs 35m

Total lap of Ireland time = 197 hours and 44 minutes

Average marathon time = 5 hours and 39 minutes

APPENDIX 2 – IMPACTS OF A STROKE[8]

Psychological and Emotional Impacts
Depression and anxiety are common. Many sufferers experience intense bouts of crying, feel hopeless, withdraw themselves from social activities and can experience a great sense of fear. Feelings of anger, frustration and bewilderment are also usual, while emotionalism, or difficulty controlling emotional responses, such as crying or laughing, scourges many. This can be extremely hard to deal with, especially in social situations, and can negatively impact relationships.

Cognitive Impacts
One or more cognitive functions can be disrupted by a stroke, such as communication, spatial awareness, memory, concentration, executive function (the ability to plan, solve problems and reason about situations) and praxis (the ability to carry out skilled physical activities, such as getting dressed or making a cup of tea).

Movement Problems
Strokes can cause weakness or paralysis on one side of the body and result in coordination and balance problems. Many survivors experience extreme tiredness and may also have difficulty sleeping. As sleep is an essential repair function of the body, its disruption stunts the healing process and can bring further health complications.

Communication Problems
Many survivors experience problems with speaking and understanding, as well as reading, spelling and writing.

Some may ultimately lose the ability to speak but can still understand what is being said to them. Common difficulties include automatic swearing, slurred or difficult to understand speech, mixing things up, like yes and no, or saying brother when meaning to say, sister. Sometimes one side of the face and tongue is paralysed or weak, and this can affect speech. This can be testing and frustrating for the stroke sufferer and disconcerting for loved ones.

Swallowing Problems
A stroke can interrupt a normal swallowing reflex, which can lead to lung damage and trigger a lung infection. Patients are often fed using a nose tube during the initial phases of recovery to prevent further complications. In the long term, exercises to improve control of the muscles involved in swallowing are required.

Visual Problems
Strokes can damage the parts of the brain that receive, process and interpret information sent by the eyes. This can result in only seeing the left or right side of what's in front of you or having double vision.

Bladder and Bowel Control
Some strokes damage the part of the brain that controls the bladder and bowel. This can result in urinary incontinence and difficulty with bowel control. This can be a short or longer-term impact.

APPENDIX 3 - REFERENCES

1.Irish Heart Foundation, 2021, Last accessed 13 March 2021, Available at: https://irishheart.ie/heart-and-stroke-conditions-a-z/stroke/

2. Intercollegiate Stroke Working Party. National clinical guideline for stroke, 5th edition. London: Royal College of Physicians, 2016.

3. American Stroke Association, 2019, Life After Stroke, Last accessed 13 March 2021, Available at:
https://www.stroke.org/-/media/stroke-files/life-after-stroke/life-after-stroke-guide_7819.pdf?la=en

4. Centers for Disease Control and Prevention, 2020, Last accessed 13 March 2021, Available at:
https://www.cdc.gov/stroke/types_of_stroke.htm

5. World Health Organisation, 2020, The top 10 causes of death, Last accessed 13 March 2021, Available at:
https://www.who.int/news-room/fact-sheets/detail/the-top-10-causes-of-death

6. Irish Heart Foundation, 2021, Last accessed 13 March 2021, Available at: https://irishheart.ie/our-mission/our-policies/stroke/

7. Stroke Association, 2017, State of the Nation, Last Accessed 13 March 2021, Available at:
https://www.stroke.org.uk/sites/default/files/state_of_the_nation_2017_final_1.pdf

8. National Health Service, 2019, Recovery Stroke, Last accessed 13 March 2021, Available at:
https://www.nhs.uk/conditions/stroke/recovery/